W9-BYJ-022

WITHDRAWN

THE JOY OF PREGNANCY

THE COMPLETE, CANDID, AND REASSURING COMPANION FOR PARENTS-TO-BE

TORI KROPP, R.N.

Foreword by Michael C. Scott, M.D.

HARVARD
COMMON
PRESS

MORE PRAISE FOR
The Joy of Pregnancy

"As both a skilled labor nurse and a popular childbirth educator, Tori Kropp has helped thousands of mothers navigate the challenges of pregnancy and delivery. She brings a wonderful combination of well-grounded practical advice and great personal insight, all done in an upbeat style. Birth is a magical experience, and I can think of no better companion to see you through."

—**Elliott Main**, M.D., Chair, Department of Obstetrics and Gynecology, California Pacific Medical Center, San Francisco

"It is with the utmost of pleasure and pride that I can finally enjoy the fruits of Tori's labor of love. Here is the most up-to-date, common-sense, honest, and complete guide for the pregnant women wishing to find all the answers to those day-to-day questions that no one, yet everyone, knows. Pregnant women need to feel they are doing the best for their unborn children, and I am confident this book can help them achieve that goal."

—**Madelyn Kahn**, OB/GYN, California Pacific Medical Center, San Francisco

"*The Joy of Pregnancy* is a must-read for all pregnant women. Tori Kropp explains the joy and wonder of being pregnant, and offers the practical advice and information women need to make the most of their pregnancies. I strongly recommend this book."

—**Will Hammett**, M.D., Central Ohio OB/GYN

"Pregnancy is an amazing and transformative experience. In *The Joy of Pregnancy*, Tori Kropp shares her own joy in this most wondrous time. This clear, calm, and reassuring guide to pregnancy will steer many women and their partners on their journeys through pregnancy and childbirth."

—**Jeanne-Marie Crowe**, C.N.M., M.S., San Francisco Women's Healthcare

More praise for Tori Kropp
from former patients and students of her
PillowTalk childbirth education classes

"I took several childbirth education classes with Tori Kropp. Her straightforward explanations and years of hands-on experience made me feel that I knew just what to expect while in labor. Her words played in my head every step of the way. Tori, you are awesome, thank you!"

—**Wendy Ficklin**, Hermosa Beach, CA

"There were so many questions my husband and I had about childbirth. I was especially worried about pain relief during labor, and Tori explained all my options so clearly I became far less worried. She was supportive, non-judgmental, and really put me at ease. She definitely made my husband feel more relaxed!"

—**Julia Peacock**, San Francisco, CA

"I have to admit that I wasn't very excited about attending my wife's childbirth class. I expected it to be too earthy and too 'touchy-feely' for me. I even brought along a stack of tennis magazines to read. I was pleasantly surprised to find Tori's class so informative and entertaining that I didn't even open one. My wife was shocked to find that I even asked several questions!"

—**Brian Muller**, Corte Madera, CA

"When Tori told us that instead of reading piles of pregnancy books we should go out to dinner and enjoy being two before we were three, I had such a sense of relief. It felt so good to just *be* pregnant instead of feeling like I had to know everything!"

—**Elaine Stoddard**, Western Springs, IL

"My husband and I benefited greatly from taking Tori's Childbirth Education class through PillowTalk. Tori's pragmatic and sensible approach to childbirth was so refreshing and helped us feel prepared and well informed when the time came to have our babies!"

—**Cristina Prescott**, Kentfield, CA

"What I appreciated most about Tori was her straightforwardness. I am a very modest person and in class she 'told it like it is' while respecting my sensitivity. During my labor and birth she helped me to feel comfortable with what my body was doing."

—**Therese Quinn**, Mill Valley, CA

"During the challenging birth of my child, a flurry of important decisions had to be made. Tori was the voice of knowledge and sensibility. We were incredibly fortunate to benefit from her medical knowledge and her acute understanding of the anxiety that faces expectant mothers. If Tori had not been there, the entire experience would have been so much more stressful and far less joyous."

—**Karen Rosenquist**, San Anselmo, CA

"When I first met Tori I was pretty adamant about not using any medications during my labor and birth. My idea of a 'natural' childbirth was 'medication free.' Once I was in labor I found that I really wanted the help of medication to ease the pain. Tori was right: 'Meds or no meds, giving birth IS natural.' All three of my babies needed to be induced and I made sure that Tori was there for all of them. She has a very calm and soothing presence about her."

—**Francesca Hetfield**, San Francisco, CA

"Tori was instrumental in the birth of our second daughter, Elle. She made us feel at ease and enabled us to take the information she had taught us and put it to real use during our birth. In fact, we were fortunate enough to have her by our side during the delivery.... She will always hold a very special place in our hearts."

—**Les Singer**, Edmond, OK

"Tori is not only my dear friend and mentor—I will always be grateful to her loving nature and expert guidance through my own labor. I will always remember the joy of being able to deliver my daughter Kate right into Tori's arms."

—**Gabriela Martinez**, Novato, CA

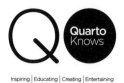

Inspiring | Educating | Creating | Entertaining

Brimming with creative inspiration, how-to projects, and useful information to enrich your everyday life, Quarto Knows is a favorite destination for those pursuing their interests and passions. Visit our site and dig deeper with our books into your area of interest: Quarto Creates, Quarto Cooks, Quarto Homes, Quarto Lives, Quarto Drives, Quarto Explores, Quarto Gifts, or Quarto Kids.

© 2018 Quarto Publishing Group USA Inc.
Text © 2008, 2018 Tori Kropp

First Published in 2018 by The Harvard Common Press, an imprint of The Quarto Group,
100 Cummings Center, Suite 265-D, Beverly, MA 01915, USA.
T (978) 282-9590 F (978) 283-2742 QuartoKnows.com

The Harvard Common Press titles are also available at discount for retail, wholesale, promotional, and bulk purchase. For details, contact the Special Sales Manager by email at specialsales@quarto.com or by mail at The Quarto Group, Attn: Special Sales Manager, 401 Second Avenue North, Suite 310, Minneapolis, MN 55401, USA.

22 21 20 19 18   2 3 4 5

ISBN: 978-1-55832-919-5

Digital edition published in 2018
eISBN: 978-1-55832-920-1

Originally found under the following Library of Congress Cataloging-in-Publication Data

Kropp, Tori.
The joy of pregnancy : the complete, candid, and reassuring companion for parents-to-be / Tori Kropp.
p. cm.
Includes index.
ISBN-13: 978-1-55832-306-3 (pbk.)
ISBN-13: 978-1-55832-305-6 (hardcover)
1. Pregnancy—Popular works. I. Title.
RG551.K76 2008
618.2—dc22   2007046213

Design: Laura H. Couallier, Laura Herrmann Design
Cover Image: Susia So
Page Layout: Claire MacMaster, barefoot art graphic design
Photography: Shutterstock.com
Technical Illustrations: Jackie Aher

Printed in China

The information in this book is for educational purposes only. It is not intended to replace the advice of a physician or medical practitioner.

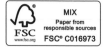

Dedication

FOR MY HUSBAND, RAYMOND B. KROPP, M.D.,
an incredible partner and father and a gifted physician
who taught everyone he knew how to live a life
of integrity, passion, and love.

AND FOR MY ALEXANDER,
whose light shines so brightly on the planet and whose
magical spirit has touched the deepest corners of my heart.

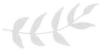

Contents

Preface

IT'S HARD TO SAY WHEN I STARTED ON THIS PREGNANCY PATH; it seems as though I have always been on it. But I recall being intrigued in high school by the plastic pelvis and the childbirth diagrams that my best friend's mom used in teaching Lamaze classes. I loved listening to Mary's mom, a maternity nurse, teach and talk about "her babies." My fascination with birth led me on a long and expanding road through the world of pregnancy. It has been 28 years since my initial enchantment, and for me, pregnancy is still more a passion than a career.

There is nothing I know more about or love more than "birthing" babies. I've helped babies come into the world in hospitals, birth centers, bedrooms, bathtubs, and hammocks, and even in the back of a pickup truck. I have seen more than 5,000 children enter the world, and birth is no less magical to me today than it was the first time. My heart warms when a woman, with a child (or two or three) in tow, makes a bee-line across the street to say, "Tori, do you remember me? You were with me eight years ago when my son was born," or "Thanks! We learned so much in your classes—they made such a difference for us." What could be more fulfilling?

So, how did *The Joy of Pregnancy* come about? Some years ago, I began to recognize that many women who had taken childbirth classes and read all the latest books on birth were coming to the hospital ill prepared for labor. Their mistake seemed to be in "thinking" their way into the experience. With so much information available, they were trusting a variety of writers and other "experts" more than they trusted themselves. They were struggling to control the very primal and uncontrollable experience of childbirth. I would sometimes spend half a woman's labor trying to help get her on track.

Women were more worried, anxious, and serious than I'd seen in the past. I wanted to understand what they were learning and why their attitudes had changed. So I began to observe childbirth classes and pore over the most popular books about pregnancy and birth. Among the best-selling books, I discovered plenty of opinions, biases toward what were deemed better "methods" of birthing, and just enough medical information to make a first-time mom worry a lot. Much of what I read was alarmist, outdated, and impractical.

Where was the humor of that expanding belly, the funny stories and old wives' tales? It seemed as though the lightness of this wonderful time was being replaced by dry facts about procedures, tests, and nutrition. I began to wonder if our mothers and grandmothers enjoyed their pregnancies more than we do today because they didn't feel the need to know so much. Information about how to take care of ourselves during pregnancy is essential, but women were getting overwhelmed.

Childbirth classes weren't much better. Instructors were trying to pass on everything they knew about having a baby, and they had sixteen hours, spread over four weeks or even a single weekend. It was simply too much. A childbirth educator myself, I presented my material in much the same way that my peers did. In my head now, I yelled, "Enough! Stop!"

I decided to make a fundamental shift in my own practice. My objective became to help women turn away from the popular approach of amassing colossal amounts of information. I wanted to become a voice of reason and common sense, with some reassuring lightheartedness. In 1990, I started my PillowTalk classes, which, within a year, were bursting at the seams. Couples were coming from 30 miles away because they had heard great things about the classes—that these sessions were "different."

The first thing I tell women in my classes is that they have some serious homework to do throughout the rest of their pregnancies. Their assignment is to stop reading a myriad of pregnancy books and instead go to the movies, have romantic dinners with their spouses, and enjoy the special anticipation of this time, before their families expand.

What I see next is very telling. It's as though a weight has been lifted. I watch the relief on their faces as they consider simply being pregnant. They have been given permission to relax and enjoy pregnancy rather than dissect it and figure it all out.

In PillowTalk classes, we talk a great deal about what each of us expects and values. Together, women learn that they each have different needs. We talk about letting go of control and about trusting—our bodies, the process of pregnancy, and the people helping us. We talk about the fact that the experience of labor and birth is neither predictable nor intellectual. We talk about choices and decisions. We talk about the fact that there isn't any one right, better, or perfect way to give birth—or, for that matter, to be a parent. The discussions validate the women's own feelings and instincts and build their confidence in themselves.

The classes also allow women to connect with one another. During pregnancy and early motherhood, women need such connection to others who are going through the same experiences. Women can connect not only by attending childbirth classes but also by joining new moms' groups and meeting at parks with their babies. In the age of cyberspace, too, we have a remarkable way to bring women together, regardless of where they live or what their daily lives are like.

With this in mind, I launched a website, Stork Site, in 1996. Stork Site quickly evolved into the largest Internet community of pregnant women and new parents. Although this was early in the life of the Internet, over 100,000 "Storkies" regularly chatted on-line about pregnancy and anything else. Being able to converse at 2:00 A.M. with another pregnant woman who says, "I know just how you feel," may seem commonplace now, when there are hundreds of pregnancy websites. But in 1996, this was an incredible new support system. Storkies even formed community networks and developed "in-person" relationships.

By sharing the experiences of pregnancy and birth through my nursing, teaching, and website, I have learned that mothers are the real experts on having babies. In 2000, I joined the moms' club myself, by giving birth to my first child, Alexander. Like every other pregnant woman, I worried about certain things and was stunned by my body's ability to adapt. Labor was and wasn't what I had expected, and motherhood is more amazing than I ever imagined.

The biggest hurdle women face in pregnancy and childbirth today, I have found, is wading through the opinions and expectations of others. My goal with *The Joy of Pregnancy* is to help you in the most nonjudgmental way possible to prepare for your babies, so that you can fully enjoy the wonders of motherhood. I have put my heart and soul into writing a book that I hope will be fresh, honest, uplifting, funny, and empowering for you as you experience your journey through pregnancy.

While I was writing this book, my life took a heart-wrenching turn. The love of my life, my husband, Ray, was diagnosed with terminal cancer. After a grueling course of chemotherapy, he died 14 weeks later. I wasn't certain I could finish the book, but knowing how happy Ray was for my opportunity to write it helped me continue. Ray was my best friend and best critic, and his strength and spirit will always guide me. *The Joy of Pregnancy* stands as a monument to his enthusiasm for the work I so love.

Come join me. I welcome you to read and learn and take from these pages anything that you find helpful. As my sweet husband said, "The ride is great. There is nothing more beautiful than a pregnant woman. Babies are unbelievable, and humor is the ingredient that keeps us sane and happy."

Acknowledgments

I GIVE SPECIAL, HEARTFELT THANKS TO THE FOLLOWING PEOPLE: Matthew and Adam, you welcomed me into your lives and have been an unwavering source of love and support. Your brilliance laid the foundation on which this book could be built. Thank you.

To Linda Konner, for being my advocate and my literary mentor, and to everyone at Harvard Common Press, especially my editor, Linda Ziedrich, and my publisher, Bruce Shaw. You believed in me from our first meetings. I have been a challenging learner—thank you for your patience and unfailing support. Thank you to Patricia Boyd for placing the sheen on the manuscript.

To my loving and creative friends, Wendy Ficklin and Tamairah Boleyn, and to the imaginative minds way back at Lot 11 Studios.

To Leslie Harlib and all those who contributed to Stork Site's content and community. I thank you for your words and creativity. Your work inspired me to write this book.

To Nicole Fainaru-Wada and Gaby Hautau, for loving PillowTalk and Stork Site, and who will forever be my very special friends.

To all my family, my sisters, and especially my mom and dad, Ernest and Magdalene Petrick. You believed in Stork Site and *The Joy of Pregnancy* when they were just ideas, and your critique, humor, advice, and love have allowed me to believe I can do anything. Special thanks to Filippa Rosenberg and Erik Hogfeldt—thank you, Filippa, for the days I barricaded myself in the "office" (AKA that special corner of the kitchen).

To my Sanity Sisters—you awesome Wednesday girls—Cris Genovese, Irene Damico, Julie Muller, Julie DeGraves, and Leslie Schuppan. We have held each other's hands since our babies were born. Now, 12 children later, you are still my most ardent fans. Thank you for holding me up when we all lost Ray, for adding your ideas to chapters, and for writing book titles on napkins. Thank you, Cris, for being my most gracious "twins" guru.

To the amazing nurses, physicians, and nurse-midwives at California Pacific Medical Center in San Francisco, with whom I have the honor to work every single day. You are my colleagues, my friends, and my family. I especially want to thank those who have most closely supported my work: Carol Abrahams, M.S., R.N.; Vicki Brumby, B.S.N.; John Fassett, M.S., C.N.M.; Bernard Gore, M.D.; Nancy Huttlinger, B.S.N., R.N.; Madelyn Kahn, M.D.; Michael Katz, M.D.; Elliot Main, M.D.; Chelan McCandless, B.S.N., R.N.C.; Hilary McGloin, R.N.; Christina Oldini, B.S.N, R.N.; and Eileen Spillane, M.A., R.N., H.N.P.

A very special thanks to William Hammett, M.D., for the time and attention you have given to the manuscript and for being a good friend.

Thank you to Maryann Barr, Ph.D., for being who you have always been to Ray and me, and to Tina Fossella, M.F.T., for honoring my heartache and for creating the space for Alexander to heal his little heart.

For John and Linda Wintermute, the best friends I could ever hope for. You have spent summer after summer living through each new phase of writing, as well as caring for and loving Alexander and me and, always, Ray.

And, finally, thanks to all the women whose pregnancies and births I have had the privilege of sharing. Forgive me if you are not listed here. You are most certainly in these pages.

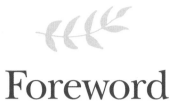

Foreword

EXPECTING A BABY should be one of the most joyous times in a woman's life. The anticipation of meeting the new life growing inside of her can fill an expectant mom with great excitement. But the journey through pregnancy also has twists and turns, hills and valleys, leaving the mom-to-be to feel anxiety, frustration, and fear, wondering about such questions as:

- What's happening to my body?
- What kinds of foods should I avoid?
- Is my baby healthy?
- What can I expect during childbirth?
- What if something goes wrong?

What do expectant parents need to know? Everything ... or so it seems. Deciding where to turn to for the answers can prove overwhelming in itself. Where do you begin? *The Joy of Pregnancy* is a comprehensive, month-by-month resource that can help every mother-to-be along her journey.

By the time you received the exciting news, you may have already picked a health-care provider to care for you and your baby throughout your pregnancy. It's important to choose someone you trust to help map out your journey; that's the first step toward making informed decisions. Prenatal visits and good daily care are important to a healthy pregnancy. When you visit your provider, listen, ask questions, and take notes.

It's also useful to find out what perinatal educational classes are available in the community. Informative classes can help make your journey more enjoyable—for you, your partner, and your baby.

As the chief of obstetrics and gynecology for the leading maternity hospital in the United States, I counsel many women each year to do their homework—to prepare themselves for the journey and for their new arrival. However, it's also just as important to experience the joy of pregnancy.

From the moment she learns she's pregnant, nearly every expectant mom is bombarded with information from her physician, family, friends, books, and the Internet. Knowledge is power, right? Not necessarily. Don't allow the information overload to overwhelm you. Relax. The stress of trying to learn it all actually can cause you and your baby some harm. Remember: You can't learn everything at once, and there is no one way or right way to experience pregnancy. Every pregnancy is unique.

Every expectant mother wishes that she had a trusted companion to hold her hand throughout her pregnancy. With this book, Tori Kropp helps by sifting through all of the information available and providing it in a practical and organized fashion, so that moms-to-be can experience the joy of their journey through pregnancy. Enjoy the ride!

Michael C. Scott, M.D., F.A.C.O.G.
Chief, Department of OB/GYN, Northside Hospital, Atlanta, Georgia

How to Use
The Joy of Pregnancy

....

THIS BOOK IS DESIGNED to make it as easy as possible for you to pilot your way through pregnancy, birth, and those first few weeks as a new mom. On these pages, you will learn about your baby and your body, and you'll find helpful ideas and strategies for dealing with the many small challenges that arise in pregnancy. Additionally, you'll read real questions from women and men like yourself, and my answers to those questions. You'll learn about my personal and professional experiences, and you'll read stories from my girlfriends and other moms with whom I have worked.

The book is organized to make it easy for you to find the information you need when you need it. There are ten chapters, one for each lunar month after pregnancy is confirmed (at two weeks after conception, or four weeks of gestational age) and one for the early postpartum period. Each topic is covered under the month in which it is most likely to be a concern. For example, morning sickness is covered in "Your First Month," which covers gestational weeks four through seven, because nausea most often begins around week six. Choosing childbirth classes and gathering baby goods are covered in "Your Sixth Month" and "Your Seventh Month," respectively, because you'll probably start thinking seriously about these things in those months. In all the chapters, I will discuss how your baby is growing, what is happening within your body, how you may be feeling, what plans you might make, and what activities might be good for you during this time. Preceding the chapters that describe each month, you'll find the brief section "Preparing for Pregnancy," which may be helpful if you are not yet pregnant. The afterword comprises inspirational stories about mothers and fathers and what they mean to their children. You can, of course, read faster than your pregnancy progresses, but by taking your time and learning as you go along, you may feel as though you have a trusted friend walking beside you. In the end, you'll feel better prepared and more confident.

You may notice that, throughout the book, I refer to the baby alternately as he and she. This is to help you identify with the material a little more easily in case you happen to know the sex of your baby.

HOW DO YOU CALCULATE YOUR DUE DATE?

Knowing when your baby will be born is one of the most baffling questions ever pondered. All right, perhaps that is a bit of an exaggeration, but nonetheless the answer can be quite confusing. Let me explain right away, so you'll understand how this book is organized.

Your due date, or *estimated date of confinement* (a very old-fashioned term!), is the approximate date that your baby will be born. The determination of this date depends on the assumption that pregnancy usually lasts about 40 weeks, or 280 days, or ten lunar months from the first day of a woman's last menstrual period. Your practitioner will use a pregnancy calendar, probably a circular one with two arrows and all the dates of a calendar year. When one arrow is placed on the date your last period began, the other will point to your estimated date of confinement (EDC). Specific markings on the calendar will indicate the approximate date you conceived (when you were two weeks pregnant, according to the calendar!) and the average weight and length of a baby conceived on that day.

Similar to the circular pregnancy calendar is the chart on pages 22 and 23, which you can use to find your own due date. Your EDC is the date directly next to the date your last menstrual period (LMP) began. Another simple way to find your EDC is to count backward three months from the first day of your last menstrual period and then add seven days.

If you have become pregnant through in-vitro fertilization, your fertility specialist will use a slightly different calendar. It calculates your EDC from the date your embryos were transferred into your uterus.

Although your EDC is a particular day, your baby will be considered full-term if he is born anytime between 37 and 42 weeks after the first day of your last menstrual period. The vast majority of babies are born within a week before or after the EDC.

Your baby's gestational age is another way of saying how many weeks pregnant you are. In this book, all references to gestational age or pregnancy weeks should be understood according to the 40-week pregnancy calendar.

Throughout the book, I will occasionally refer to the first, second, and third trimesters of pregnancy as well as pregnancy weeks and months. Each trimester is about three months on a regular calendar, or about 13 weeks.

Find Your Due Date

LMP = January	1	2	3	4	5	6	7	8	9	10	11	12	13	14
EDC = October	8	9	10	11	12	13	14	15	16	17	18	19	20	21
LMP = February	1	2	3	4	5	6	7	8	9	10	11	12	13	14
EDC = November	8	9	10	11	12	13	14	15	16	17	18	19	20	21
LMP = March	1	2	3	4	5	6	7	8	9	10	11	12	13	14
EDC = December	6	7	8	9	10	11	12	13	14	15	16	17	18	19
LMP = April	1	2	3	4	5	6	7	8	9	10	11	12	13	14
EDC = January	6	7	8	9	10	11	12	13	14	15	16	17	18	19
LMP = May	1	2	3	4	5	6	7	8	9	10	11	12	13	14
EDC = February	5	6	7	8	9	10	11	12	13	14	15	16	17	18
LMP = June	1	2	3	4	5	6	7	8	9	10	11	12	13	14
EDC = March	8	9	10	11	12	13	14	15	16	17	18	19	20	21
LMP = July	1	2	3	4	5	6	7	8	9	10	11	12	13	14
EDC = April	7	8	9	10	11	12	13	14	15	16	17	18	19	20
LMP = August	1	2	3	4	5	6	7	8	9	10	11	12	13	14
EDC = May	8	9	10	11	12	13	14	15	16	17	18	19	20	21
LMP = September	1	2	3	4	5	6	7	8	9	10	11	12	13	14
EDC = June	8	9	10	11	12	13	14	15	16	17	18	19	20	21
LMP = October	1	2	3	4	5	6	7	8	9	10	11	12	13	14
EDC = July	8	9	10	11	12	13	14	15	16	17	18	19	20	21
LMP = November	1	2	3	4	5	6	7	8	9	10	11	12	13	14
EDC = August	8	9	10	11	12	13	14	15	16	17	18	19	20	21
LMP = December	1	2	3	4	5	6	7	8	9	10	11	12	13	14
EDC = September	7	8	9	10	11	12	13	14	15	16	17	18	19	20

LMP means the first day of your last menstrual period.

Use the first day of your last menstrual period (LMP) to find your estimated date of confinement (EDC)

15	16	17	18	19	20	21	22	23	24	25	26	27	28	29	30	31
22	23	24	25	26	27	28	29	30	31	1	2	3	4	5	6	7

15	16	17	18	19	20	21	22	23	24	25	26	27	28
22	23	24	25	26	27	28	29	30	1	2	3	4	5

15	16	17	18	19	20	21	22	23	24	25	26	27	28	29	30	31
20	21	22	23	24	25	26	27	28	29	30	31	1	2	3	4	5

15	16	17	18	19	20	21	22	23	24	25	26	27	28	29	30
20	21	22	23	24	25	26	27	28	29	30	31	1	2	3	4

15	16	17	18	19	20	21	22	23	24	25	26	27	28	29	30	31
19	20	21	22	23	24	25	26	27	28	1	2	3	4	5	6	7

15	16	17	18	19	20	21	22	23	24	25	26	27	28	29	30
22	23	24	25	26	27	28	29	30	31	1	2	3	4	5	6

15	16	17	18	19	20	21	22	23	24	25	26	27	28	29	30	31
21	22	23	24	25	26	27	28	29	30	1	2	3	4	5	6	7

15	16	17	18	19	20	21	22	23	24	25	26	27	28	29	30	31
22	23	24	25	26	27	28	29	30	31	1	2	3	4	5	6	7

15	16	17	18	19	20	21	22	23	24	25	26	27	28	29	30
22	23	24	25	26	27	28	29	30	1	2	3	4	5	6	7

15	16	17	18	19	20	21	22	23	24	25	26	27	28	29	30	31
22	23	24	25	26	27	28	29	30	31	1	2	3	4	5	6	7

15	16	17	18	19	20	21	22	23	24	25	26	27	28	29	30
22	23	24	25	26	27	28	29	30	31	1	2	3	4	5	6

15	16	17	18	19	20	21	22	23	24	25	26	27	28	29	30	31
21	22	23	24	25	26	27	28	29	30	1	2	3	4	5	6	7

EDC means your due date.

Becoming Pregnant

IF YOU'RE TRYING TO GET PREGNANT or thinking about trying, I recommend that you see your practitioner for a preconception visit. This can take place during your annual well-woman exam, that is, the gynecological checkup in which you have a general health assessment, a manual breast exam, and, often, a Pap smear. Let the office know ahead of time that you'd like to include a preconception discussion, so that time will be allotted for it.

Your doctor or nurse-practitioner will take a Pap smear if you haven't had one done within the past year or two. A Pap smear is a swab of cervical tissue taken during a pelvic exam and analyzed for irregularities. Treating a cervical problem identified through an abnormal Pap smear is easier before pregnancy than during it.

Make sure all your vaccinations are current. Because I never had chicken pox (varicella) as a child, and because I am around children a lot and know that chicken pox in pregnancy can be dangerous to the baby, I chose to receive the varicella vaccine before attempting a pregnancy.

As part of the exam, your practitioner will review any medical condition you may have and may also check for others. You may have a blood test for possible conditions. Let your doctor or nurse-practitioner know how you are feeling, if you have any chronic medical problems, if you take any medications, and if you have had any significant changes in your health or your life recently. A problem such as depression, diabetes, hypertension, or a thyroid or autoimmune disorder should be reviewed, and the treatment "tuned up," to help ensure the best outcome for your pregnancy. A medication that you take might need to be switched to one considered safer during pregnancy. Your practitioner may recommend that you have any needed dental work or medical tests, such as an X-ray or a cardiac evaluation, before you get pregnant, when these procedures may be easier and sometimes safer.

Although it's best to maintain good health all the time, you'll want to take excellent care of yourself as soon as you stop using birth control. Be conscientious about eating healthful foods, staying fit, and maintaining or working toward your ideal weight.

Women's health practitioners now routinely recommend that all women of childbearing age take a multivitamin that includes at least 400 micrograms of folic acid. A deficiency in folic acid has been shown to be responsible for the birth defect spina bifida. Folic acid intake before pregnancy may be more important than intake after conception, perhaps because the nutrient needs to build up at the cellular level. For this reason, many practitioners recommend that a woman take a prenatal multivitamin containing folic acid for at least three months before trying to get pregnant. Prenatal multivitamins, many of which are available without a prescription, all contain the vitamins and minerals essential before pregnancy, during pregnancy, and for breastfeeding. Unless your practitioner recommends a particular one, you can choose whichever you like.

If you drink beverages containing caffeine or alcohol, you may want to stop or decrease your intake before becoming pregnant. Some recent research has shown that women who consume more than 300 milligrams of caffeine daily take longer to become pregnant than those who consume less caffeine or none. Although an occasional alcoholic drink doesn't seem to affect fertility, some studies have found that the probability of conception in a particular menstrual cycle decreases as a woman's alcohol intake increases, even among women having five or fewer drinks per week.

After you stop using birth control, how long might it take you to get pregnant? This depends partially on your age. Biologically, the ideal time for women to be pregnant is from our late teens through our early thirties. As we become older, our balance of reproductive hormones changes, and it becomes more difficult for us to conceive and to maintain a healthy pregnancy. Today, unlike 20 years ago and very unlike 40 years ago, women are tending to have babies later in life. Most women becoming pregnant in the United States are 25 to 35 years old. Most professional women becoming pregnant are 30 to 35 years old. In the past ten years, the rate of pregnancy in women over 35 has increased by 30 percent. Mature women feel more settled and better prepared for parenthood, and that is good for their children. But fertility rates decrease with advancing age, and after age 40, on average, they drop sharply. With continual advances in assisting fertility, more and more women over age 40 are having babies. In the United States in 2015, the birth rate for women in their 40s was 10.6 per 1,000

When Ray and I were married, I was 34, and we wanted to have a family "within a couple of years." Two years later, my doctor suggested that we needed to think seriously about getting started. Like many of my friends, I had assumed that I would become pregnant whenever Ray and I decided that we were ready. Well, when I was 37, we finally felt ready, but I did not become pregnant. After a year and a half of trying to conceive, I learned that my hormones were already in the perimenopausal range. With each passing month, my chances of getting pregnant were diminishing. Alexander was born when I was 39, and we were very fortunate to have him.

The decline of fertility varies from one woman to another. There is no critical change that happens when a woman turns 35. If you have not conceived after six months to a year of actively trying, the American College of Obstetricians and Gynecologists suggests that you be checked by your practitioner. "Actively trying" means not just having intercourse now and then but also using a natural method of ovulation prediction and timing.

Ovulation occurs when at least one mature egg is released from one of your ovaries into the fallopian tube on the same side. Your highest chance of becoming pregnant occurs if you have intercourse from one to two days before ovulation to approximately 24 hours afterward.

Specific signs can help you determine your most fertile time. By paying close attention to your body over a few months, you can learn to identify the signs of approaching ovulation.

Cervical mucus. As you near ovulation and the level of estrogen in your body rises, your body produces more mucus, which becomes clearer and more slippery than earlier in your cycle. This change in the texture of your cervical mucus helps sperm travel up through your cervix and into one of your fallopian tubes.

Rise in body temperature. After ovulation, your temperature will increase between ½ and 1 degree Fahrenheit. You can detect this increase in one of two ways. First, you can find your basal body temperature by taking your temperature at the same time every morning. The release of an egg stimulates the production of the hormone progesterone, which raises your body temperature. A spike in temperature indicates that you have ovulated. Your temperature varies naturally depending on the time of day and what you are doing, so variations in how and when you take your temperature can make it hard to identify the small increase that follows ovulation.

A second way to measure the rise in your body temperature is by using an ovulation predictor kit. You can use the kit to check your urine for luteinizing hormone, which surges just before ovulation. Ovulation predictor kits are easier to use and are considered more accurate than the basal body temperature method. Because these kits can predict ovulation 12 to 36 hours in advance, you can maximize your chance of conception from the very first month that you use them. The kits are readily available, without a prescription, in drugstores and supermarkets.

Lower abdominal discomfort. One woman in five feels an ache, a cramp, or a twinge on one side of her lower abdomen at the time of ovulation. This pain, called *mittelschmerz,* can last from a few minutes to two hours.

If these natural methods don't work for you, see your doctor or nurse-practitioner. General obstetrician-gynecologists successfully treat most infertility problems. Depending on your particular situation, your doctor may recommend that you see a fertility specialist or reproductive endocrinologist. These doctors work only with infertility, of all types. A single visit can provide you with a wealth of information regarding tests and treatments that may be appropriate and available for you.

I wish the very best for you on your journey to motherhood.

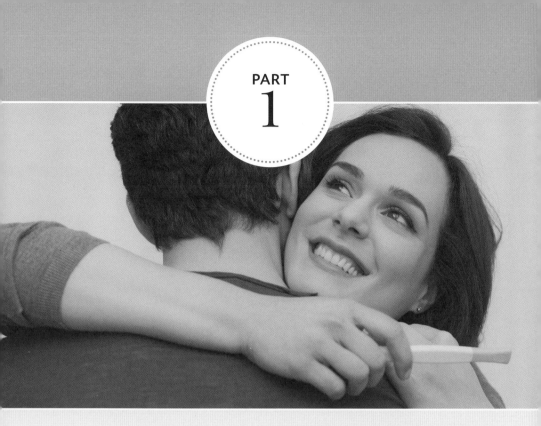

THE FIRST TRIMESTER

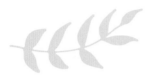

Enter Your Amazing Pregnancy!
YOUR FIRST MONTH: WEEKS 4 THROUGH 7

CONGRATULATIONS—YOU'RE PREGNANT! You have probably just missed your menstrual period or have confirmed your pregnancy with a home urine test or with a blood test taken by your practitioner. These things happen at approximately week four of pregnancy, which on the gestational calendar begins month one.

You may not feel any different physically yet, but your emotions may be stirring. Happiness, ambivalence, excitement, fear, anxiety, and joy are some of the emotions you will experience over these next nine mysterious and wonderful months. All these feelings are a normal part of becoming a parent.

One of the most important things I have learned about birthing babies is that the process is more of an unfolding marvel than a routine progression of events. Much of the time, the various aspects of pregnancy and birth are predictable. But pregnancies vary. Some women experience nausea, some have extreme fatigue, and others, like my friend Julie, find that flowers smell sweeter and the world looks brighter while they are pregnant. Some women feel mostly challenged by pregnancy, and others mostly delighted, but the vast majority feel both these emotions almost equally during pregnancy.

The normal variations from one pregnant woman to the next can be confusing when you are looking for answers and reassurance. Your best friend's pregnancy may be very different from yours, and comparing the two pregnancies may not be helpful at all. My goal is to help you understand the many physical and emotional changes you will experience during your pregnancy. As you read this book, you will recognize that your experiences are normal—that many other pregnant women are feeling the same way you are. I want you to get comfortable with all the changes you experience.

Now let's talk about what's happening within your body and how your very tiny baby is growing.

WHAT'S HAPPENING WITH YOUR BABY?

You may remember the first time that a grade-school or junior-high health or science teacher outlined for you how conception occurs. Although many of us learn about the physiology of conception early in life, we may not think about the details until we try to become pregnant or actually are pregnant.

Here is a basic review of the process. An egg, or more than one, is released by one of a woman's ovaries and travels down through one of the fallopian tubes. When a man ejaculates during lovemaking, semen is deposited into the woman's vagina. Within the semen are millions of sperm, which, aided by the woman's slippery cervical mucus, travel into and through the woman's cervix. Many of the sperm continue through the uterus and up the fallopian tube to the egg. As soon as one sperm penetrates the egg, the egg and sperm unite. Within hours, the fertilized egg cell begins to divide, and the egg travels from the fallopian tube into the uterus. In a few days, the fertilized egg will attach itself to the wall of the uterus, and the placenta will begin to form.

Your baby grows very rapidly. At week four, she is approximately ¼ inch long, about the size of a pea, and looks a lot like a tadpole. At this stage, she is still called an embryo. During weeks four through six, her neural tube forms; it will later develop into the baby's brain and spinal cord. Your baby's body has small limb buds, which will later develop into her arms and legs. She is beginning to show signs of a face, and her organs are developing rapidly. She has a beating heart. Using an ultrasound machine with an amplifier, you and your practitioner will probably be able to both see and hear your baby's heartbeat by week six.

WHAT'S HAPPENING WITH YOUR BODY?

Even though your body has been going through many changes for the preceding two weeks, week four is when you will first be able to confirm that you are pregnant. Home pregnancy tests are widely available and quite accurate. Many can show a positive result in as little as four days after your menstrual period is due. The tests work by detecting in your urine the pregnancy hormone *hCG* (human chorionic gonadotropin), which is produced by the developing placenta and released into your bloodstream. To take the test, you simply hold the test stick in the stream of urine while you are peeing. If the result is positive, the stick will change color within one minute. It's a good idea to perform the test the first thing in the morning, when your urine is likely to be the most concentrated. If you are pregnant, your first urine in the morning probably has the highest concentration of hCG.

The home pregnancy test is a qualitative, not quantitative, test; that is, it tells you *whether* hCG is present in your urine, but not *how much* hCG is present. For the test to show a positive result, there must be a certain minimum amount of hCG in your urine. An "early result" pregnancy test is designed to detect a lower amount of hCG. For example, if the test has a minimum detectable amount of 50 milli International Units (mIU) per milliliter, the result will be positive only if your level is higher than 50 mIU. Four days after your period is due, your hCG level might be only 48 mIU, and so the test result might be negative even if you are pregnant. But hCG levels rise daily, and three days later, your level might be 140. If you tested again, the result would be positive. As you can see, women who test early sometimes show a negative result even though they are pregnant. For this reason, most tests come two to a package. If you take an early pregnancy test and get a negative result, but your period hasn't started two weeks after it was due, be sure to repeat the test.

A blood test for pregnancy is quantitative; that is, it measures the actual amount of hCG in your blood system. This test can show a positive pregnancy result 14 days after conception. If you have received medical assistance in becoming pregnant, such as artificial insemination, ovarian stimulation, or in-vitro fertilization, your doctor will want you to have two blood tests two to three days apart, to monitor the rise in hCG.

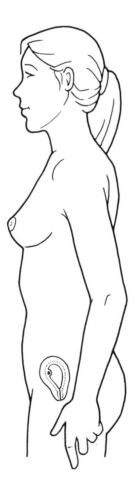

Normal hCG Levels in Pregnancy

Time from Conception	Gestational Week	hCG Level (mIU/ml)
7 days	3	5–50
21 days	5	18–7,340
28 days	6	1,080–56,500
35–42 days	7–8	7,650–229,000
43–64 days	9–12	25,700–288,000
57–78 days	13–16	13,300–254,000
second trimester	17–24	4,060–165,400
third trimester	25–40	3,640–117,000

The chart "Normal hCG Levels in Pregnancy" outlines the expected rise in hCG levels through pregnancy. As you can see, normal levels vary greatly. Women who are pregnant with twins or triplets have higher levels, but even women pregnant with single babies have greatly varying hCG levels. The important thing is that your level should double every two to three days in early pregnancy. Levels peak at about eight to ten weeks, steadily decline until the third trimester, and then remain at the lower level for the remainder of the pregnancy.

IMPORTANT THINGS TO KNOW

Regardless of how you discovered that you were pregnant, there are many ways this little growing being is letting you know that he is there.

Signs and Symptoms of Pregnancy

It is normal to have some, all, or none of these symptoms. Although some of the signs can be annoying, keep in mind that these symptoms are also an indication that your hormones are flowing as they should, and that your body is responding to its greatest change of all.

SLIGHT BLEEDING OR A BROWNISH VAGINAL DISCHARGE ABOUT TWO WEEKS AFTER CONCEPTION

This is usually caused by the implantation of the fertilized egg (the *blastocyst*) in the uterus. Sometimes, a woman may mistake this implantation bleeding for her menstrual period. Even if you have what seems like a light period, you may still be pregnant.

NAUSEA, WITH OR WITHOUT VOMITING

"Morning sickness," which can occur at any time of day, is thought to be caused by the increase in the hormone hCG, which is produced by the placenta. Nausea is the most common early sign of pregnancy. It generally starts at about six weeks, when the level of hCG rises most significantly. If you have not been closely tracking your menstrual cycle, nausea may be your first clue that you are pregnant. We'll talk more about coping with morning sickness later in this chapter.

MORE FREQUENT URINATION

Your uterus is beginning to grow. Even though the change is small, the growth causes pressure against your bladder. Some women notice this more than others do.

SLEEPINESS

I can't tell you how many times I have heard moms say, "I slept my way through my pregnancy." Sleepiness is a very common sign of pregnancy. Before you were pregnant, you may have often felt sleepy at some point during the day but pressed on with your work anyhow. Now you may find that however you try, you cannot deny your body the rest it needs. Hormones are largely responsible, especially the rise in your body's production of progesterone. Your body is using more energy, too, for the hard work of growing a baby. Extra sleep is not a luxury now; it is a necessity. The good news is that sleepiness declines after the first trimester.

DIZZINESS OR LIGHTHEADEDNESS

During pregnancy, all your organs and systems undergo dramatic changes. The most significant changes occur within your cardiovascular system. To meet the increased metabolic needs of your baby, several things happen. The amount of blood circulating in your body increases by 40 to 50 percent, reaching a maximum volume at approximately 32 to 34 weeks. Your circulatory system supplies your uterus and your baby with the nutrients needed for growth. Most of the added blood volume is in your uterine, placental, and breast tissue.

Your heart begins to beat faster to pump more blood per minute throughout your body. In the early weeks, your blood pressure gradually decreases, reaching its lowest point in the middle of your pregnancy. It then begins to rise, and by the end of pregnancy, it returns to its normal level.

Low blood pressure can cause you to feel dizzy or lightheaded. This is most noticeable when you get up quickly from a lying or sitting position. Standing too quickly moves blood away from your brain, which makes you feel lightheaded. This is quite normal and nothing to worry about. The feeling is most common during the early months.

When you feel lightheaded, be careful to move a little more slowly and to hold on to a chair, the wall, or another stable object for support and balance. This is especially important when you are getting out of the shower or bath. In warm water or a hot room, your blood vessels dilate, lowering your blood pressure.

Try not to sit or stand in one place for too long. When you sit or stand for more than a few minutes, blood pools in your feet and lower legs. If you stand up suddenly, your blood may not return to your heart from your legs fast enough. As a result, your blood pressure may drop quickly and you may feel faint.

Exercising your calves will increase the circulation in your legs. Occasionally stretching your legs, marching in place, rolling your ankles in a circular motion, or walking (even short distances) throughout the day will help keep your blood circulating well.

Another good habit to start now is to roll onto your side before rising out of bed. Besides helping to prevent lightheadedness, this practice will protect your abdominal muscles from strain as your belly becomes larger.

When you feel lightheaded, sit down or squat and put your head between your knees. This will help move blood up into your head and make you feel better.

Lightheadedness from low blood pressure usually passes in the second trimester. Be aware, though, that low blood sugar, or hypoglycemia, can also cause dizziness. Your nutritional needs are greater now that you are pregnant, and you need to eat plenty of healthy food. Having frequent small daily meals rather than three large ones will help keep your blood sugar stable. Carry healthy snacks with you when you're away from home so that you can eat whenever you get hungry.

Dizziness can also be caused by anemia, or a deficiency of iron in the blood. The increase in blood volume can cause a decrease in the concentration of hemoglobin (red blood cells) circulating through your body. If you are anemic, you have fewer red blood cells to carry oxygen to your brain and other organs, and you may feel weak, tired, and dizzy. For this reason, it is important to maintain an iron-rich diet and to take a prenatal multivitamin that includes iron (see page 80). Your practitioner will check your hemoglobin level through an initial set of blood tests. If you are anemic, he or she may suggest adding an iron supplement to your prenatal multivitamin. Don't take extra iron unless you truly are anemic, because iron can be constipating and upsetting to the stomach.

Is It Really Necessary to Drink Six to Eight Glasses of Water a Day?

During pregnancy, your increased energy needs, faster metabolism, and hormonal changes alter your body's physiology. You also have an increased blood volume, and your baby is producing amniotic fluid. All these changes require your body to have more water than usual.

It's not possible to know exactly how much water each of us should drink each day. Remembering to drink a minimum number of glasses, however, is a simple way to prevent dehydration. I suggest drinking six to eight glasses a day, plus one or two more if you exercise or it is a hot day. A good way to know if you are well hydrated is that your urine will be a very pale yellow.

CONSTIPATION

This can be a problem even if you don't take iron supplements. Many women feel constipated in the first trimester because of the rise in progesterone, which can slow the process of passing bowel movements. Increasing your fluid intake, exercising regularly, and increasing the fiber in your diet are some of the ways to prevent or minimize constipation.

If you're a big water drinker, staying well hydrated won't be hard. If not, you'll have to begin a new habit and try to stick with it. Many women add a thin slice of lemon, orange, cucumber, or other refreshing fruit to spiff up their water. A little lemon did the trick for me.

You will also want to eat a variety of high-fiber foods—fruits, vegetables (especially peas and beans), and whole grains. Nuts and seeds also contain fiber but have a higher fat content, so eat them in moderation.

A variety of herbal tea blends marketed for pregnancy correct or prevent constipation, or both. I recommend that you discuss with your practitioner any medicinal herb you'd like to use, even if the product is sold in the supermarket.

If you experience constipation after increasing your fluid and fiber intake, ask your practitioner about the stool softener docusate sodium. It is sold over the counter and is considered safe for pregnancy.

UNUSUAL HUNGER OR FOOD CRAVINGS

These are caused by two things: hormonal changes similar to those you may have experienced during your menstrual cycle, and your body's need for extra nutrients to support your growing baby. Indulging in these cravings is a good, fun way to increase your nutrition during pregnancy.

DARKENING OF YOUR AREOLA

This darkening of the pink or brown area around each nipple is due to an increase in pregnancy hormones and is part of your body's preparations for breastfeeding your baby. You may also notice a darkened line extending from your navel to your pubic hairline. This *linea negra*, as it is formally called, also results from hormonal increases.

SWOLLEN AND TENDER BREASTS

During pregnancy, many women feel tenderness down the sides of the breasts and a tingling or soreness in the nipples. The growth of the milk-producing lobules and the ducts that carry the milk to the nipple can cause this discomfort in the breasts. Although you may notice swelling and tenderness earlier, they are more pronounced after six weeks.

GENITAL CHANGES

Your labia, the lips of your vulva, may darken and feel a little swollen, and you may notice more colorless vaginal discharge than usual. These changes will probably increase during your second and third trimesters, when your estrogen levels will rise.

Clean Living

If you planned your pregnancy for some time, you may have already changed some habits that might be harmful to your baby. If not, you may need to make some lifestyle changes now.

Please don't worry if, before you knew you were pregnant, you did something you'd rather you hadn't. This is true for many women, and very seldom is any harm done in these cases. But you may be consuming or otherwise using certain things that you should now stop using altogether, cut down on, leave to someone else to deal with, or use only with caution. Run a mental check on the following products.

CIGARETTES: Stop.

Cigarette smoke contains nicotine, tar, and carbon monoxide, all of which are toxins that prevent oxygen from getting into your bloodstream and passing on to your baby. If you smoke, placental blood flow is constricted and your baby receives less nutrition. Babies whose mothers smoke are born smaller, on average, and have a higher chance of being born prematurely and having later learning disabilities. Both placenta previa (a condition in which the placenta is implanted low in the uterus and covers all or part of the cervix) and placental abruption (the premature separation of the placenta from the wall of the uterus) are twice as common among smokers as among nonsmokers. There is a higher incidence of Sudden Infant Death Syndrome (SIDS) among babies exposed to cigarette smoke.

In the mother, of course, smoking can cause emphysema, cancer, and a multitude of other health problems. Remember, your family needs you.

Quitting on your own can be very difficult. If you need help, talk with your practitioner about strategies. Among the possibilities, smoking-cessation support groups have shown the highest rate of success. You can probably find such a group at your local hospital or community center.

What Is Sudden Infant Death Syndrome (SIDS)?

SIDS is defined as the sudden, unexplained death of an infant younger than one year old. The majority of SIDS deaths occur when babies are between two months and four months old. In 2015, the rate of SIDS was approximately 1 death per 2,000 babies. The cause of this syndrome is unknown, and the diagnosis is made when all other possible causes of death have been ruled out. It is responsible for far fewer deaths than congenital disorders and disorders related to pre-term birth. Despite the lack of specific knowledge about why some babies succumb to SIDS, the incidence of the syndrome has declined over the last two decades. The American Academy of Pediatrics continues to recommend that healthy babies be placed on their backs to sleep. The national "Back to Sleep" campaign, initiated in 1994, provides extensive education to new families about infant sleep positions.

Breathing secondhand smoke can be nearly as dangerous as smoking. If your partner smokes, ask him to do it outside or at least away from you. This could be a good time for him to work on quitting.

ALCOHOL AND ILLEGAL DRUGS: Stop.
Everything you ingest crosses the placenta. This includes alcohol and drugs.

Exactly how much alcohol is needed to harm a fetus is unknown, but some studies have found an increased risk of miscarriage, premature labor, and birth abnormalities with two glasses of wine per day. Alcoholic mothers give birth to babies with Fetal Alcohol Syndrome, which includes numerous physical and mental abnormalities resulting from brain damage caused by maternal drinking. Fortunately, there appear to be no negative effects on babies from brief periods of heavy drinking in early pregnancy.

Among illegal drugs, marijuana is the most common used today. Smoking marijuana before getting pregnant or soon afterward has not been shown to harm a baby, but there is evidence that continued marijuana use affects the function of the placenta and may result in a baby's low birth weight. A baby of a marijuana smoker is more likely than other babies to experience fetal distress during labor. Additionally, the newborn baby may experience withdrawal symptoms such as jitters, poor response to stimuli, and problems latching on to the breast and sucking. Neurobehavioral, verbal, and memory defects that show up in children after age three or four may also be associated with marijuana use in pregnancy.

The effects of marijuana on a woman and her pregnancy are also significant. Women who smoke marijuana regularly are likely to have poor nutritional habits. Although marijuana can cause an increase in appetite, the foods selected are often not healthy. Women who smoke marijuana are more likely than other women to have preterm labor and precipitous (extremely rapid) labor.

Stimulant drugs such as cocaine and methamphetamine can be devastating to the developing fetus. Children exposed to cocaine in the womb are more likely to have symptoms of attention-deficit hyperactivity disorder (ADHD), which include impulsivity, distractibility, and certain learning deficits. Animal studies suggest that prenatal exposure to methamphetamine may have adverse developmental effects, although we don't yet know exactly what these effects are or how long they may last.

A mother's use of opiods, intravenous narcotics, and heroin do not appear to have as severe an effect on a developing baby as the stimulant drugs do. Still, use of these drugs can harm a mother's general health and her ability to care for her children. It is very important to know that babies go through significant withdrawal from any mood-altering drug that the mother has taken during her pregnancy.

Parents who use any illegal drugs also risk having their children taken away from them. If you are having trouble giving up any drug, I encourage you to talk with someone who can help you—your practitioner, a counselor, or even a friend. Many women have changed their lives because of their babies, and you can, too.

CAFFEINE: Stop or cut down.

This stimulant crosses the placenta; when you have a cup of coffee, so does your baby. Caffeine also causes blood vessel constriction, which at least theoretically affects the baby, too. The many studies on caffeine and pregnancy have produced confusing results. The general recommendation, however, is that pregnant women should have no more than one daily serving of a beverage or food containing caffeine.

Many women find even the smell of coffee nauseating during pregnancy. Some, though, have a tough time either giving up or cutting down on this beverage. Decaf coffee can be a very tasty substitute, and most processors use safe, natural methods to decaffeinate the beans. If you must have the real thing, try to limit yourself to one cup a day.

Remember that tea, chocolate, and many sodas also contain caffeine.

FISH: Be aware.

Fish and shellfish are valuable components of a healthy diet; they are rich in protein and contain omega-3 fatty acids (page 87), which can help prevent heart disease. The richest sources of omega-3 fatty acids are oily, cold-water fish, including large fish such as swordfish and shark.

The larger and older the fish, unfortunately, the more pollutants such as mercury they contain. Mercury occurs naturally in the environment and is released into the air through industrial pollution. Over time, this metal accumulates in streams and oceans and is absorbed by fish. Recent increases in pollution of our waters limit how much of this wonderful food we should eat. The amount of mercury we get from food isn't thought to be harmful for most people, but high levels of mercury could affect your baby's developing nervous system. The same is true for PCBs (polychlorinated biphenyls), industrial chemicals also found in certain fish and shellfish.

Generally, ocean fish are safer than lake fish. The U.S. Food and Drug Administration recommends that you not eat swordfish, king mackerel, bluefish, striped bass, American eel, or shark during pregnancy. Shrimp, light canned tuna, salmon, and catfish generally contain low levels of mercury and are considered safe to eat. Different kinds of lake fish are affected in different regions. Your practitioner may be able to give you specific recommendations for safe eating. You can find a wealth of helpful information from the Monterey Bay Aquarium's excellent program Seafood Watch, www.mbayaq.org/cr/seafoodwatch.asp.

CHEESE: Be aware.

Has someone told you that you shouldn't eat "soft cheese" during your pregnancy? This is only partly true. Some ripened soft cheeses, such as Brie, Camembert, and blue-veined types, can harbor the pathogen *Listeria*, which is found in water and soil. *Listeria* primarily affects pregnant women, newborns, and adults with weakened immune systems. It causes extreme sickness in the mother and can cause a miscarriage or premature delivery. A baby who becomes infected may die before or shortly after birth.

Although the incidence of infection is extremely low, pregnant women are advised not to eat such cheeses. Since cooking kills *Listeria*, baked Brie would be fine. Hard or semihard cheeses such as cheddar and Monterey jack are also safe. So are soft, fresh, pasteurized cheeses such as cottage cheese and cream cheese and processed cheese products in sealed packages. Queso fresco, a moist and crumbly cheese that is often sprinkled over enchiladas, black bean soup, and salads, is fine as long as it is pasteurized.

All cheese should be kept chilled, and fresh cheeses should be eaten while fresh.

CAT LITTER: Be aware; have someone else change it.

Many women follow this good advice without knowing why. The problem isn't with cat litter itself; it's with an organism called *Toxoplasma gondii*, which is sometimes found in cat feces and which can cause the infection toxoplasmosis. Early in your pregnancy, when you have your first set of blood tests, your practitioner may test you for antibodies to toxoplasmosis. If your practitioner doesn't do the test routinely, you can ask for it. If you have owned a cat or eaten raw meat in the past, you may have already been infected with toxoplasmosis. In a child or an adult with a healthy immune system, this generally asymptomatic infection causes no harm. If you have never been infected, however, you are at some risk of developing an initial infection during pregnancy. In this case, your baby would be infected, too. A small proportion of infected infants develop visual disabilities, brain damage, mental retardation, and seizures.

The likelihood of getting an infection during pregnancy is very low, but if you lack antibodies to *Toxoplasma gondii*, you will want to take some simple precautions. Stay away from raw-meat dishes, such as carpaccio and steak tartare, because raw or undercooked meat can harbor the organism. If possible, have someone else clean the cat's litter box. If this isn't possible, use disposable liners in the litter box, or wear rubber gloves and wash your hands well with warm water and soap after cleaning or changing the litter.

If you are a gardener, wear gloves while digging in the dirt. Scrub your hands and nails when you are done, especially if you know that cats sometimes visit your garden.

CLEANING PRODUCTS AND SOLVENTS: Be aware; have someone else apply them.

As we have all become more aware of the effects of cleaning products on our environment, it has become easier to find nontoxic products. You can find effective "green" cleaning products in natural-food stores, in mail-order catalogs, and on the Internet; many supermarkets now carry them, too. Switching to safe cleaning products is a great way to begin creating a healthier environment for your family.

You can generally assume that a cleaning product is safe unless there is a warning label on the package. If you are not sure of a product's safety, wear gloves and work in a well-ventilated area. Women sometimes find the smells of cleaning products bothersome during pregnancy, and fresh air can help with that problem, too.

It's normal to want to freshen up a home before your baby's arrival. If you decide to take on a renovation project, be the organizer and director, and leave the dirty work to your mate or another designated person. You shouldn't clean with solvents, strip paint, or do any painting while you are pregnant.

LEAD: Be aware.

Exposure to lead is particularly dangerous before and during pregnancy. Lead poisoning can occur in adults, but this heavy metal is most dangerous to unborn and very young children, whose brains and nervous systems are in the early stages of development. Lead stays in the body a long time, so exposure is cumulative.

Lead in the environment comes from many sources, including paint, old pipes, solder, and ceramic and pewter cookware. Because paint on the walls and woodwork of houses built before 1980 may have a high lead content, any stripping or sanding of these painted surfaces may release lead dust into the air. Old pipes may contain lead, and so may some modern faucets and the solder in lead-free pipes (although new building codes require lead-free solder). Products made outside the United States, including toys, may also contain lead. Any lead in municipal water supplies is removed at the treatment plant, but water can become contaminated with lead in household plumbing, and private well water can contain lead as well as other contaminants. It's best to have your tap water tested for safety early in your pregnancy, if not before. If you do have lead in your household plumbing, it's a good idea to let the water run for a minute or so the first thing in the morn-

Bottled water isn't necessarily any healthier than municipally supplied tap water. Both must meet the same standards of purity.

ing to flush out the water that's been sitting overnight in the household pipes (you can save this water for watering your houseplants). And always start out with cold tap water, not hot, for cooking. Water from hot-water tanks contains more minerals and can dissolve lead from the pipes more readily than cold water does.

X-RAYS: Be aware.

With today's equipment, the risk of X-ray overexposure is extremely small. Still, it's best not to have an X-ray during pregnancy unless you really need one, such as for a broken bone. In this case, all precautions will be taken to ensure your own safety and that of your baby. X-rays are also used in dental care, but generally not during pregnancy. If you must have a dental X-ray, you and your baby will be protected with a lead shield.

If You're Not Feeling Well: Morning Sickness

One of the most unpleasant symptoms of pregnancy is intermittent nausea, vomiting, or both. Some women are far more affected than others. Those who have experienced motion sickness are somewhat more likely to have morning sickness. The good news is that for most women, the symptom subsides by the end of the first trimester, or by 12 to 14 weeks. I have several tricks in my bag for helping you cope with the minor discomforts of morning sickness.

Drink plenty of fluids. Vomiting can cause dehydration, which can be harmful to you and your baby. But sometimes drinking causes more vomiting. Fruit juices, such as apple or orange, can be upsetting to the stomach, especially when it is empty. Drinking too much at once or too quickly may be counterproductive, too. Try drinking fluids between meals instead of with them to keep from feeling too full. If you have been vomiting, you can try an electrolyte drink such as Gatorade. These drinks shouldn't be your main source of fluids, though; they are too high in sodium, potassium, and sugar.

If drinking anything at all nauseates you, try a variety of things that melt into liquid, such as Jell-O. Ice pops are terrific, too; the cold is refreshing. You can find healthy frozen juice bars in stores or make your own. But if an ordinary sugar ice pop is the only thing you can keep down, then that's exactly what you should have!

Carbonated drinks such as colas and ginger ale are frequently soothing to the stomach. Even though cola may contain caffeine, having an occasional cola is fine if it helps curb your nausea.

Eat smaller, more frequent meals, five to six a day. Low blood sugar increases nausea. Carry with you healthy and appealing snacks, such as crackers, popcorn, and cheese slices. Eat before you get really hungry.

Eat something even before you get out of bed in the morning, if necessary. Plain crackers work well for many women. Ice pops worked for me. I had pretty dreadful morning sickness when I was pregnant with Alexander. Every morning, Ray brought me a plain orange ice pop, which I ate before I even raised my head. That little bit of cold fluid and sugar helped me start my day.

Morning Sickness Does Not Occur Just in the Morning.

Nausea can hit at any time of the day. It tends to be worse, though, when a woman has an empty stomach and low blood sugar. This condition occurs most often after a night's sleep.

Eat anything that appeals to you, including milk shakes, ice cream, pasta, or other high-calorie foods. You want to eat as healthily as you can, of course, but if you are really having trouble with nausea and food aversions, you'll need to temporarily alter your nutritional habits. Unless you are very overweight and your practitioner recommends that you not gain any additional weight, you should gain about 3 to 8 pounds (1.4 to 3.6 kg) during the first trimester. If instead you aren't gaining at all or are even losing weight, the rule of thumb is calories, calories, calories. If you are not taking in enough for both you and your baby, you will be the one who goes without. But I'm not giving you license to eat cartons of ice cream and cookies throughout pregnancy. Once your nausea has passed, move on to foods that are more balanced.

Tori's Tip: Be Good to Yourself

If you have morning sickness, don't expect yourself to "tough it out." Ask for help from those around you. You and your baby are the most important people in your world right now.

Stay away from spicy or fried foods and smells that make you queasy. It is fair to ask your spouse not to indulge in that big plate of greasy onion rings right in front of you. And if you're bothered by smells from cooking, the garbage can, coffee, dirty dishwater, cleaning products, or scented toiletries, stay away from them.

Take your prenatal multivitamin with your largest meal. Even without morning sickness, vitamins can upset your stomach. If indigestion is a problem, you might want to try a multivitamin that includes a stool softener, stomach antacid, or both. If you have trouble swallowing a large pill, you might prefer a chewable multivitamin. Ask your practitioner what he or she recommends.

Mint tea and the smell of a freshly cut lemon can help.

Try to slow down. Getting enough sleep, relaxing more, and decreasing your stress level can lessen nausea, too.

Change the way you brush your teeth. If the taste of your toothpaste bothers you, try switching to a more natural brand. If it's the act of brushing that makes you gag, brush quickly and gently, and do not brush your tongue; you can follow up with a good mouth rinse. If your teeth or gums are sensitive, look for toothpastes labeled for sensitive teeth. Your dentist or dental hygienist may have some good recommendations.

Try motion-sickness bands. These come in two types, both of which are completely safe. The first is a small elastic band that applies pressure to an acupressure point on the inner wrist, about two finger-widths away from the base of the hand. This type costs about $6 to $10 per pair and is available at marine and dive shops and pharmacies. The second type is battery-powered and looks like a wristwatch. It emits a small pulse, delivering mild electrical stimulation to the nerves in the inner wrist. Although the device didn't work for me, I know many moms who swear by it. The biggest drawback is the cost, $85 to $100. The device is available in some stores and over the Internet. If your practitioner prescribes the device for morning sickness, your insurance company may reimburse you for the cost.

Acupuncture has been shown to decrease nausea in pregnancy.

Fresh air can do wonders. Try sleeping with a window open, sitting outside, or taking a walk.

Severe morning sickness—the inability to keep any food or liquid down—is called *hyperemesis* (from *hyper,* "over," and *emesis,* "vomiting"). Dehydration is the most common serious side effect of hyperemesis. If you are unable to keep down any food or liquid, are losing weight, or are dizzy or faint throughout the day, contact your practitioner right away. Occasionally a woman with hyperemesis needs to be hospitalized briefly and rehydrated with intravenous fluids.

When Something Goes Wrong

Although there may be very good medical explanations for why a woman miscarries or has other problems that end her pregnancy, the emotional pain can be very real. But a look at why things can happen, and the reassurance that these difficulties are rare and seldom prevent a woman from having a successful pregnancy later, can help reassure a woman and her partner.

MISCARRIAGE

A miscarriage happens when an embryo or a fetus dies or a pregnancy fails for another reason. Most miscarriages, or spontaneous abortions, as they are also known, result from random chromosomal abnormalities of the embryo and occur before the 8th week. Hormonal irregularities, vaginal infections, poorly controlled diabetes, thyroid disease, and lupus can add to the risk of miscarriage. Age is also a factor in miscarriage; the rate rises at around age 35. In general, the miscarriage danger zone ends at 12 to 13 weeks, as 80 percent of miscarriages happen during the first trimester.

Approximately 15 to 20 percent of confirmed pregnancies end in miscarriage. No one knows how many women miscarry before their pregnancies are confirmed or even suspected. Because of this unknown, the total miscarriage rate is probably much higher than 15 to 20 percent.

If an ultrasound scan at six to seven weeks doesn't find a heartbeat, there very well may never have been an embryo, just *trophoblastic* tissue (tissue that would have provided nutrition for the embryo). Another possibility is a *blighted ovum*, which occurs when a fertilized egg attaches itself to the uterine wall and cells develop to form the pregnancy sac but not the embryo. This problem, which causes about half of first-trimester miscarriages, is chromosomal. It can be caused by abnormal cell division or a defect in the sperm or egg.

Second-trimester miscarriages are unusual. They may be caused by a maternal health condition or a problem with the uterus, such as an abnormal shape, fibroids (noncancerous growths in the uterine wall), or a weakened, or "incompetent," cervix that dilates prematurely.

An incompetent cervix is the cause of nearly 25 percent of second-trimester miscarriages (or 1 percent of all pregnancies). This problem can result from cervical surgery, cervical trauma, or a genetic defect. Although an incompetent cervix is usually diagnosed after a second-trimester miscarriage or a preterm delivery, a procedure called cerclage can prevent the cervix from opening prematurely in a subsequent pregnancy. Cerclage is most commonly performed, under general or spinal anesthesia, between 12 and 14 weeks, but it can also be done as an emergency measure in the second trimester. A woman is often placed on bed rest after a cerclage (see page 176).

The initial signs of miscarriage can be subtle. You may notice brownish or reddish spotting that becomes heavier over a few days. First-trimester bleeding can be normal—a benign sign of the embryo's implantation in the uterus (between weeks four and five) or the increase in capillaries in the cervix. Miscarriage brings additional symptoms. You may no longer feel pregnant. Your breasts may no longer be tender, or you may feel less nauseated or tired. If you are miscarrying, these symptoms will progress.

A Woman Doesn't Cause Her Miscarriage.

Women who miscarry often wonder, "Could I have done something to prevent this?" Absolutely not. It's important to take the best possible care of yourself before and during pregnancy, but you cannot control acts of nature.

Severe cramping, with or without bleeding, is the most definitive sign of an impending miscarriage. Mild cramping is common during the first trimester of a healthy pregnancy, but severe cramping is not. Constant cramps that are painful enough to keep you from carrying on daily activities are a sign of trouble.

When a pregnancy ends, the body initiates uterine contractions to expel the fetal and placental tissue, and bleeding occurs. If you miscarry early in your pregnancy, you may not yet have seen your practitioner for your first prenatal visit. Whether or not you have had this first visit, your practitioner may now ask you to wait at home for further symptoms before seeing you. There is nothing he or she can do to stop a miscarriage.

If you miscarry once, you have an excellent chance of carrying the next baby to term. A woman who has had a single first-trimester miscarriage for no known cause is at no added risk of having a subsequent miscarriage.

Even a woman who has had two consecutive miscarriages has good odds the third time around; chances are two out of three that she'll carry her next baby to term. If you miscarry twice, though, you may want to have tests done to rule out any other causes besides random chromosomal abnormalities. After the results are in, your practitioner can discuss with you any particular risk of future miscarriages and can suggest possible preventive treatments.

After a loss, you may wonder how long to wait before trying for another pregnancy. Many practitioners recommend waiting through one normal menstrual cycle so that the body can recover and return to normal. Studies show, however, that a pregnancy that begins immediately after a miscarriage is at no higher risk than one that starts later. You may want to wait, anyway, perhaps longer than one cycle, until you feel emotionally ready to try again.

Whether or not you start trying to get pregnant again right away, you will probably grieve. The time needed to heal from a loss is very individual. You will probably feel worse if people make insensitive comments such as "It was for the best" or "You are young; you can try again." These kinds of comments are not meant to be hurtful. Death is an uncomfortable topic for many people, some of whom don't understand how a woman can grieve the loss of a person she never met. Your partner may not share your depth of grief, or he may feel just as sad but not show it. Try to find supportive people among your family or friends, or join a support group of others who have miscarried. Check with your practitioner or a local hospital for help in locating one.

When you get pregnant after miscarrying, you may worry a lot, especially during the danger zone of the first 12 or 13 weeks. Please know that your anxiety is normal and likely to fade as your pregnancy moves along.

For more on miscarriage, see page 51.

ECTOPIC PREGNANCY

In an ectopic pregnancy, the embryo grows outside the uterus, most commonly in one of the fallopian tubes. Although the embryo may be healthy, the pregnancy cannot continue. If the embryo continues to grow, it will rupture the fallopian tube and threaten the mother's life.

In the U.S. population, a little more than 1 percent of pregnancies are ectopic. The rate has increased over the years, very likely because of an increase in tubal infections, or *salpingitis*, caused by gonorrhea or chlamydia. Other risk factors are previous tubal surgery, reversal of tubal sterilization, and the use of an intrauterine device (IUD) at conception. But ectopic pregnancies often happen to women with none of these risk factors.

Early symptoms of an ectopic pregnancy are subtle. They can include crampy pain occurring approximately two to four weeks after the last menstrual period (gestational weeks six to eight), possibly on only one side of the pelvis; light bleeding or spotting, either brownish or reddish; low back pain; and nausea.

If an ectopic pregnancy isn't treated before rupture begins, the symptoms become severe. The woman may feel intense lower abdominal pain, which may decrease or cease abruptly when the tube ruptures and then begins radiating to the neck, shoulder, or back. Other likely symptoms are dizziness, weakness, and fainting; nausea and vomiting; and shock. *If you have any of these symptoms, you need to be taken to a hospital for immediate surgery.*

If suspected early, an ectopic pregnancy can be diagnosed through blood tests and an ultrasound scan. A doctor will check the level of hCG (human chorionic gonadotropin) and then repeat the test in two to three days. If the level is high enough to suggest pregnancy but is not increasing normally, either an ectopic pregnancy or a miscarriage may be the cause. An ultrasound scan can confirm an ectopic pregnancy.

An ectopic pregnancy that is diagnosed early may sometimes be treated without surgery. The mother is given an injection of methotrexate, a drug approved by the U.S. Food and Drug Administration (FDA) for the treatment of certain chronic diseases and cancers. Methotrexate stops the growth of the embryonic and placental cells and induces the passage of the embryo and placenta.

In many cases, laparoscopic surgery is necessary. With this technique, the physician makes small incisions into the abdomen and inserts a small camera and surgical instruments, which are used to remove the tissue.

After an ectopic pregnancy, it is quite possible to get pregnant again safely, provided you have at least one healthy fallopian tube.

Maternity Medical Coverage

If you have not done so already, now is the time to check on your medical insurance coverage. You'll want to determine what kind of coverage you have for your pregnancy, the birth, and the new baby. You might set up an appointment with the benefits coordinator at your company or your partner's. If you are self-employed, you might call your insurance company's customer-service number.

These questions will help you get started:

- Does your plan cover prenatal and maternity care? Federal law requires that an employer with more than 15 employees offer such coverage.
- Do you need "preauthorization" from the insurance company for prenatal or maternity care? Do you need to contact the health insurance company when you're admitted to the hospital or birth center?
- Do you need a referral from your primary-care doctor to see an obstetrician? Can you make the obstetrician your primary-care doctor?
- Will your plan cover care from a nurse-midwife?
- What are the plan's policies regarding in-network and out-of-network health-care providers?
- What is the coverage for prenatal lab tests, diagnostic studies, ultrasounds, and amniocentesis?
- Does the plan cover medications that may be needed during your pregnancy?
- Does your plan require that you give birth at a particular hospital? If so, you'll want to be certain that your physician or midwife practices there.
- Will your plan cover birth at a birth center or at home?
- Do you have a deductible? If so, how much of it has already been met? Is there a separate deductible for pregnancy?
- Is there a copayment for office visits? If so, how much is it?
- How long a stay in a hospital or birth center does the plan cover? How many days are allowed for a cesarean birth and a vaginal birth? Will the plan cover an extended stay if it is medically necessary?
- After your baby is born, do you need to alert the insurance company immediately, before going home from the hospital or birth center? Many companies automatically provide coverage for a newborn if she is added to the plan within 30 days of birth.

- Which local pediatricians are within the plan's network?
- Does the plan cover your baby's hospital stay? What if the baby needs intensive care?
- Does the plan cover well-baby checkups and vaccinations? Will you have a copayment, and if so, what will it be?

If you lose or quit your job, or if your spouse does, be very aware of how your insurance coverage may be affected. If you are switching to a new company, there may be a waiting period before your new benefits begin, and your care provider and choice of birth-place may not be covered under the new plan. It can be very hard to switch practitioners midway through your pregnancy. Thanks to the COBRA Act of 1985, you can stay on your former company's health insurance plan for between 18 and 36 months if you have been fired, laid off, or given a decrease in work hours or status that would otherwise cause you to lose your benefits.

Ask Tori, R.N.

RUBELLA (GERMAN MEASLES)

Hi, Tori!

I am 28 years old and in my seventh week of pregnancy. I have just received the results from my initial blood tests, and I am alarmed to find out that I am not immune to rubella (German measles), even though I was vaccinated for it as a child. I have read that I should stay away from children and babies, as they may not have been immunized.

What are the symptoms of rubella? Is it similar to the measles? How dangerous is it to my baby, and does the risk diminish after a certain time? Must I really avoid all exposure to children?

—Elizabeth, Montana

Dear Elizabeth,

Approximately 14 percent of women lack immunity to rubella, or German measles. Although the disease is almost unknown in the United States today, rubella could cause serious problems for your baby if you were to contract the illness during your pregnancy, especially during the first three months. A rubella infection in the first trimester can cause birth defects such as deafness, blindness, heart defects, and mental retardation. After the first trimester, the danger of such effects lessens.

Talk with your practitioner about whether you need to avoid being around children. In the United States, most children are vaccinated against rubella. The MMR (measles, mumps, rubella) vaccine is usually given as two shots, the first at 12 to 15 months and the second at four to six years.

Symptoms of rubella are general malaise, swollen glands, a fever, and a rash over much of the body. If you have these symptoms, you should certainly see your doctor.

Assuming you don't contract rubella during pregnancy, talk with your practitioner about receiving the vaccine as soon as possible after you give birth. The rubella vaccine is considered safe during breastfeeding.

ALCOHOL

Tori,

This is my first pregnancy and I am concerned about the alcohol I consumed before I found out that I was pregnant. What are the possible effects, and how can I keep myself from worrying so much?

—Jessica, New Mexico

Dear Jessica,

Many women have had small or moderate amounts of alcohol or have taken medication before discovering that they were pregnant. Your baby is very likely to be completely healthy. Drinking prior to pregnancy, or having an occasional glass of wine during pregnancy (no more than two per week), has not been shown to have any adverse effects on a baby. You can limit your worrying by not drinking at all. Worry only takes away the joy of being pregnant, and you certainly don't want you to miss that. Talk with your practitioner if you need further reassurance.

MEDICATIONS FOR NAUSEA IN PREGNANCY

Tori,

I am in my eighth week of pregnancy (my first one!). I have severe nausea and vomiting. It got to the point last week that I could not keep anything down for several days. I finally saw my doctor, who said I was very dehydrated and needed to go into the hospital for intravenous fluids. When I asked him if there was any other option, he said he could give me the IV medication, Zofran, in the form of a pill.

I am very concerned about taking these pills, although they do help me tremendously and my doctor says they are safe for pregnancy. This medication is primarily used to alleviate the symptoms caused by chemotherapy treatment in cancer patients. Have you ever heard of this drug's being prescribed to pregnant women? Without it, I am unable to keep any food down at all.

—Megan, Wisconsin

Dear Megan,

When a woman has serious nausea in pregnancy, her practitioner will generally prescribe a medication that can help alleviate the symptoms. Zofran, or ondansetron, is the most useful one I've seen in my own practice. This medication is used after surgeries and chemotherapy and in cases of severe motion sickness, and I have seen many pregnant women helped enormously by it. I myself had severe nausea in early pregnancy, and I took Zofran from about 6 to 14 weeks.

Unfortunately, Zofran is costly, so some doctors and midwives have women try something else first. Phenergan, Reglan, and Compazine can be helpful for milder nausea. You may need to work with your insurance company to have payment authorized for Zofran.

You are right to want to avoid taking unnecessary medications. When you can't keep food or liquid down, however, taking medication on your doctor's advice is the responsible thing to do. It can make a big difference in your health and your baby's. If Zofran works for you, the benefits far outweigh any potential risks.

For more about medications, see page 81.

SAUNAS AND HOT TUBS

Hi, Tori,

Is it safe to visit the sauna (including steam room, hot tub, and cold-water bath) when I'm pregnant? My nurse-midwife says that it's okay as long as it feels good, but I remember reading something to the contrary.

—Sydney, Vermont

Sydney,

Although some European studies show that pregnant women can regularly soak in hot tubs or enjoy an occasional sauna without any apparent harm, most practitioners in the United States worry about the high temperatures of a hot tub or sauna. Being in the hot water or steam will increase your body temperature. A significant elevation in your temperature (over 102° F [39° C]) can be potentially harmful to your growing fetus, whether the cause is a sauna, a hot tub, an illness, or exercise. A hot bath or shower is fine as long as you keep the temperature comfortable to the touch (less than 102° F [39° C]) and finish up before you become overheated.

MISCARRIAGE

Hi, Tori,

I'm 35 and have suffered two miscarriages this year. These have been my only pregnancies. I was six weeks along when I miscarried the first time and eight weeks with the second. Now I can't stop questioning myself, and I'm terrified that it will happen again. I've been told that it was nature's way, that the baby could not have survived, and so on. But this doesn't ease my fears. How can I find out what caused these miscarriages?

—Belinda, Alabama

Belinda,

Miscarriage is one of the most heartbreaking experiences a woman can go through. Having two is particularly difficult. Although people mean well when they say that miscarriage is nature's way, this doesn't acknowledge the magnitude of your loss or validate your sadness.

Try not to blame yourself. Women often say things like "I had a glass of wine," or "We were moving, and I lifted a few boxes." A miscarriage can happen for any number of reasons, none of which are within your control.

Causes of miscarriage can't always be found, but since you have had two consecutive losses, your doctor will probably be willing to evaluate your hormone levels, conduct tests to rule out genetic factors, or take both steps. Hormonal and endocrine problems can frequently be treated with medications, either injections or suppositories. Structural abnormalities, which sometimes cause second-trimester miscarriages, can often be diagnosed and treated surgically. Unlike even 15 or 20 years ago, medical advances can now help a woman who otherwise couldn't achieve and maintain a healthy pregnancy.

SUSHI

Tori,

My friends tell me not to eat sushi, but my doctor says it is fine as long as it comes from a high-quality source. What do you think?

—Rachel, Washington

Rachel,

Practitioners whose opinions I value greatly have widely differing positions on the safety of eating sushi during pregnancy. The concern is that raw fish can contain parasites such as liver flukes and other microbes that can make you very ill. The most common recommendation is that eating sushi is fine if it contains cooked fish or shellfish or vegetables only. Many forms of raw fish are likely to be safe, however, if the fish has been properly handled. Raw fish for sushi or sashimi must be kept well iced, separated from other fish, cut with a clean knife and board, and used promptly. Once sliced, the fish should be served and eaten immediately. You can't be certain that a particular fish is free of harmful microbes, but you should at least make sure that your fish comes from a reputable restaurant or shop.

DAD'S CORNER

Amazing, isn't it? One day you are just cruising along as usual, and the next day, you are going to be a father! You may have been alerted by her dashing to the bathroom at three, five, and seven o'clock in the morning, or by the changing color of a pregnancy test stick, or even by a call from her doctor. This pregnancy may be a surprise, or it might be what you two have been working toward for months. In any case, there is no doubt that pregnancy changes things. Every new dad-to-be has certain similar experiences.

The News. Now that your partner is pregnant, do you tell everyone you know, or do you wait to see how the first few weeks or months go? For couples who have postponed having children, the tide of thrilled relatives and acquaintances can be a bit overwhelming. Many times, grandparents-, uncles-, and aunts-to-be are more excited about the prospect than are the parents. A new grandmother-to-be whom I know was so thrilled with the news that she immediately sent her daughter two sets of embroidered booties, one pink, one blue.

The Reality. Now that that your partner is expecting, it is usual and expected for you and her to feel a full range of emotions. You may feel quietly joyous or deeply ambivalent. Even though your child is just a tiny embryo, you may suddenly be worried about what kind of parent you will be. Go easy! Try to give yourself time to absorb all this change, without judging or criticizing yourself. The best way to sort out your reactions is to let yourself have them. Reading this book, at your own pace, will help you learn all about pregnancy and babies. Talk with a few friends if you like, but don't feel you have to go into an information-gathering frenzy. Most important of all may be spending time with your spouse as both of you adjust to the idea of parenthood.

Treat Her Well. Doing something special for your partner shows that you are thinking of her and of what she's going through, and that you want to be a part of it. For each month, I'll suggest a few tried-and-true gems. Here are some for month one:

Dad, "We" Aren't Pregnant.

Always keep in mind that, although you are intimately involved in supporting your partner through pregnancy and birth, she is having an experience different from yours. Acknowledging this shows respect for her hard work of growing the baby.

- Surprise her with some flowers "just because."
- Offer to take over the grocery shopping, especially if she is sensitive to smells.
- Take out the garbage and empty the cat litter box before she asks.
- Encourage her to sleep as much as she feels she needs to.

As you learn about all the different pieces in this puzzle of pregnancy, remember that one day, in the not-so-distant future, you will be holding your very own, very special baby. At each step of the journey, I hope to share insight and reassurance with you. No·matter what, one thing is certain: Your baby will be uniquely yours.

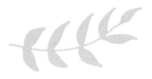

Choices and Cravings
YOUR SECOND MONTH: WEEKS 8 THROUGH 11

WELCOME TO YOUR SECOND MONTH OF PREGNANCY, the month of two new aspects of your life: choices and cravings! Every month entails choices, but in the second month, most expectant parents look for answers to their key questions, not the least of which is "Where can I get some gluten-free chocolate-anchovy pancakes?"

All joking aside, this is a time to make some important decisions. You are probably starting to think about what matters to you in your prenatal and maternity care, and your preferences will continue to evolve as you move through your pregnancy. This month, you will need to choose your care provider and think about where you would like to deliver your baby. Let's get started.

WHAT'S HAPPENING WITH YOUR BABY?

At the start of this second month, you are eight weeks pregnant, and your baby's gestational age is therefore eight weeks, too. He weighs approximately 1 gram and is about 4 centimeters, or 1½ inches, long—about the size of a small apricot. His heart is beating 60 to 70 times per minute, and his tiny vertebrae have developed. His brain, spinal cord, kidneys, stomach, intestines, liver, muscles, bones, and skin are also

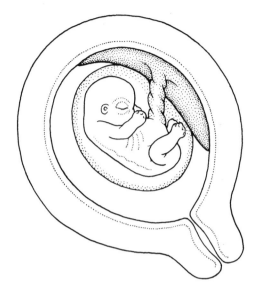

rapidly developing. They will be visible now if you have an ultrasound scan (the image is called a *sonogram*; see page 96). Your baby has facial features and well-defined ears, ankles, and wrists. On the sonogram, you will be able to see the placenta working and identify his eyelids, which are formed but sealed shut. The baby's fingers and toes are taking shape. He is no longer called an embryo but is now called a fetus. He looks more like a baby than he did last month.

WHAT'S HAPPENING WITH YOUR BODY?

Physiologically, your body is rapidly responding to the changes of pregnancy. Most of these changes are occurring within your uterus and cervix. Although you cannot feel these changes, your cervix and uterus are softening, and your uterus is shifting from its pre-pregnant pearlike shape to a more globular shape. Your blood volume is increasing, and more blood flow is being directed to your uterus.

Many of the early signs and symptoms we talked about in the preceding chapter are beginning to appear. You don't look pregnant, but you definitely are starting to feel pregnant.

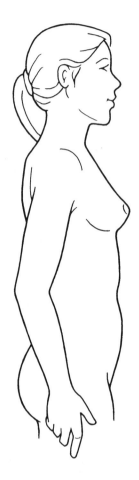

IMPORTANT THINGS TO KNOW

Even though you don't look pregnant and might still be getting used to the idea that this is happening to your body, you do need to start on some practical homework. Your growing baby knows what to do, but the sooner you are set up with your health-care team, the sooner you can relax and know that you are doing the best thing for you and your child.

Choosing a Birthplace: Hospital, Birth Center, or Home

In the United States, approximately 97 percent of women give birth in hospitals. Home births account for about 1 percent of the nation's total

Choose the Right Birthplace for Multiples

Multiple births are generally more risky than single births. Moms de-livering twins or higher-order multiples are more likely to have their babies by cesarean section, at an estimated rate of about 50 percent. Multiple births should take place at a hospital so that an operating room can be quickly available if needed. In my experience, a woman who is having twins or triplets labors in a regular, comfortable labor room and then moves into an operating room for the actual birth. This allows the doctor to be prepared should any complications arise during the birth. Because twins often come early, their parents should choose a hospital with a level 2 or 3 nursery (see below). If you are carrying twins and live far from such a hospital, consult with your doctor about what to do if you go into preterm labor.

Here is a summary of the different types of nurseries. Level 1 hospitals are generally community hospitals that care for moms with uncomplicated pregnancies giving birth at or very near full-term (35 weeks' gestation or later). Level 2 hospitals can care for a more complicated pregnancy, a high-risk labor, and babies born after approximately 32 weeks' gestation. Many level 2 hospitals have a neonatologist (high-risk infant doctor) on staff and a special nursery for smaller babies. A level 3 hospital has a neonatal intensive-care unit (NICU) that can care for the smallest babies and the most complicated births. Delivering at a hospital that has a level 2 or 3 nursery will ensure that you and your babies stay together after birth if complications arise. I strongly recommend taking a tour of the hospital you will have your babies in, before the birth, so that you will know what to expect.

births. In the mid-1980s, out-of-hospital birth centers became popular, but they are currently on the decline, partly because over the past 10 to 15 years, most hospitals have created warm, friendly maternity units with homelike, comfortable rooms.

In hospitals today, a woman can usually give birth in the same room in which she labors and can have anyone she chooses with her. Even in the most tranquil hospital room, though, medical equipment is readily available. It can be reassuring to know that, should a problem arise, the resources to handle it quickly are right there. Women who choose to give birth in a hospital say they do it for the safety of mother and baby, for support during labor, and for the opportunity to use anesthesia and other medications during labor.

Some women choose to give birth at home. Women I know who choose home birth say they want an unhurried, natural labor, free from unnecessary medical interventions. If something goes seriously wrong during labor at home, however, the mother must be transferred to a hospital. A suitable hospital must be fairly close to home. Few physicians attend these births; most home births are attended by midwives, who also provide prenatal care. The midwife must work with a physician at a hospital to which the mother can be transferred in an emergency.

Birth centers aim to provide an experience like home birth but with the guarantee of quick transfer to a hospital in case of emergency. One or more midwives or a physician is present to support the mother through much of her labor. Birth centers are generally within a hospital complex or very nearby. The center may or may not provide prenatal care on site.

There can be advantages and disadvantages to delivering in a certain setting. Advocates of hospital and nonhospital birth disagree about which is better or safer. Does hospital birth bring the possibility of increased interventions? Yes. Can it also be a wonderful experience, with plenty of support and intimacy? Yes. I have shared birth with women in all types of settings, and I have seen difficult experiences and magical ones in each. I work with women in a hospital because

I believe that a woman has more choices about the kind of birth she wishes within that setting.

In making your decision about where to give birth, take the time to think through what feels the most supportive and comfortable for *you*.

Choosing a Doctor or Midwife

You will probably have your first prenatal visit somewhere between seven and nine weeks' gestation. If you haven't yet chosen someone else to attend the birth, this visit may be with your regular obstetrician-gynecologist, nurse-practitioner, gynecologist, or family-practice physician. If you are selecting a new doctor or nurse-midwife, you may have to wait a few weeks for the first prenatal appointment. Often, the appointment is set for nine weeks into your pregnancy.

If you don't yet know who will care for you in your pregnancy, your first task may be to sort through job titles and their meanings. Most hospital births are attended by obstetrician-gynecologists; some gynecologists, however, do not practice as obstetricians. Formerly, most family-practice doctors attended births, but many have stopped because of the high cost of malpractice insurance. Nurse-midwives attend approximately 8 percent of hospital deliveries, and some attend birth-center and home births. Other home-birth midwives may be described with a variety of terms. Nurse-practitioners work with physicians and frequently help provide prenatal care, but they do not attend births.

Let me outline the basic differences among birth practitioners:

Obstetrician-gynecologists (OB-GYNs). These medical doctors specialize in the reproductive care of women. After medical school, OB-GYNs complete four years of specialized education and training in obstetrics and gynecology, including surgery.

Family practitioners. These medical doctors specialize in family medicine, which may include pregnancy and birth. After medical school, their training involves all aspects of general medical care for adults and children. Family practitioners care for women during normal pregnancies and deliveries, and for the babies.

Certified nurse-midwives (CNMs). These birth practitioners are registered nurses who have earned a graduate degree in nurse-midwifery.

The graduate program involves specialized training in caring for women during pregnancy, labor, and the weeks after birth. CNMs work with healthy women who have normal pregnancies and labors. Should a medical problem arise, a CNM consults with a backup physician.

Direct-entry, empirical, or lay midwives. These terms all refer to midwives who have entered the profession directly, through study and apprenticeship, without becoming nurses first. A *certified professional midwife* has passed rigorous tests and has received a certificate from the North American Registry of Midwives (NARM). Several states license direct-entry midwives; other states do not. Direct-entry midwives provide prenatal care for healthy women and attend normal births in homes and in out-of-hospital birth centers.

Finding the right practitioner can be a daunting task. Your regular practitioner may recommend someone, and you can ask your friends for suggestions or search the phone book for possibilities. Some large clinics provide formal assistance in choosing from their practitioners, and hospital labor nurses may provide recommendations. You may need to select a provider who is covered by your insurance plan, which may also limit your choice of birth setting. Before scheduling an appointment, you'll want to find out where the practitioner attends births and confirm that he or she works with your insurance company.

Every woman is unique in what she needs and expects from her health-care provider. As you collect referrals, consider these questions:

- Is your personal style suited to someone formal and businesslike, or would you prefer someone who runs a smaller practice and who will spend a lot of time with you?

- Would you feel more comfortable with a woman or a man, or does the person's sex not really matter to you? (I must mention that some of the most sensitive physicians I know are men. Also, I work with one of the only male nurse-midwives in the country, and he is in high demand!)

- How important is it to you that the same person who provides your prenatal care also attends your baby's birth? If your practitioner is in a group practice of doctors or midwives who alternate the times they are responsible for night or weekend births, any member of the group may end up as your birth attendant. If a nurse-practitioner provides your prenatal care, an obstetrician will attend the birth. If you choose a midwife but face complications in pregnancy or labor, your midwife may refer you to a backup physician.

- What kind of birth experience do you want? For example, do you want an unmedicated delivery, or do you think you'll want an epidural? You'll want a practitioner who has assisted other couples through the same kind of birth experience.

It is important that you feel comfortable with the philosophy of your chosen practitioner and confident in his or her skills. In talking with many women, I have found that the most important aspect of the relationship between a pregnant or laboring woman and her practitioner is trust. Whether a woman has an unmedicated birth, an epidural, or an unplanned cesarean birth makes little difference in how good she ultimately feels about the experience. The important thing is whether she felt trust in her providers and in the care she received.

To help establish this trust from the start, you might ask your prospective doctor or midwife some of these questions:

- How long is a typical office visit?
- How many births does the practitioner, or group of practitioners, manage each month?
- What are the practitioner's feelings and practices regarding fetal monitoring, epidurals, and other medications in labor? How about episiotomy, cesarean birth, and breast-feeding?
- In what situations does the practitioner induce labor? Is labor routinely induced if it doesn't begin spontaneously before 41 or 42 weeks?
- What percentage of the practitioner's patients give birth by cesarean? What is the cesarean rate for the entire practice?

- At what point in labor does the practitioner arrive?
- If the practitioner is a doctor, does the practice include certified nurse-midwives?
- Will you meet everyone in a group practice before the baby is born?
- If you have a question or a problem, how do you reach the doctor or midwife?

Many doctors and midwives are too busy to provide personal interviews before a first exam, but some of your questions can be answered on the phone. Your first prenatal visit will be the time to ask the rest of your questions. I recommend writing them down before your visit. The conversation should help you decide if this is the right practitioner for you—if you feel confident in his or her qualifications and abilities, and if he or she will provide the kind and degree of support you would like. If you decide that this practitioner isn't right for you, it will still be early enough in your pregnancy to make a change.

Choosing a Hospital or Birth Center

If your insurance plan and choice of practitioner allow you to choose between two or more birth facilities, you may want to tour each of them. You may even want to tour facilities before choosing a practitioner, and then pick a doctor or midwife who practices at the hospital or birth center you prefer. Here are some questions for you to consider:

- How far is the facility from your home?
- Is one-on-one care provided throughout labor? What is the nurse-to-patient ratio?
- Are there CNMs (certified nurse-midwives) on staff?
- Who is allowed to be with you in labor? During the birth itself? What if you have a cesarean birth?
- Are there any policies regarding the use of independent doulas (labor-support persons)?
- Will you give birth in the same room that you labor in? Can you look at the rooms?

- Does the facility have policies about the use of medical procedures such as fetal monitoring (intermittent or continuous) and the administration of intravenous (IV) fluids, or does the individual practitioner determine when and how these procedures are used?

- Will you be allowed to move about freely during labor?

Tori's Tip: Avoid Delays at Prenatal Appointments

Are you a busy woman? To get into and out of your practitioner's office as quickly as possible, schedule your prenatal appointments first thing in the morning or right after lunch. At these times, delays are less likely and your practitioner will probably be less hurried.

- Do the rooms have showers, whirlpool baths, or other bathtubs?

- Will you be allowed to eat and drink during labor?

- Is there an anesthesiologist on staff at all times?

- Is epidural anesthesia (page 298) available? Is there any restriction on when you can receive it?

- What is the epidural rate?

- Will the baby be able to stay in your room after the birth, or will the baby be taken to a nursery?

- Can you see the operating room where cesareans are performed? If you have a cesarean, can the baby stay with you afterward?

- What is the cesarean rate?

- If you or the baby requires special care, can both of you stay at the facility, or will you be transferred to another hospital?

- Does the hospital have a neonatal intensive-care unit (NICU)? If so, what level of care does it provide?

- What is the policy on breastfeeding? Can you specify that the baby not receive bottles of formula or sugar water?

- Is there a lactation consultant on staff?
- Does the hospital or birth center offer prenatal and parenting classes? Are there new-parent support groups?

Identifying what is essential to you will help you select the birth facility that is right for you. What's more, by becoming familiar with the facility on your tour, you may feel more at ease when the time comes for your delivery.

Your First Prenatal Visit

During your first visit, your practitioner will not only answer your questions but also ask *you* questions, administer some tests, and examine you. He or she will ask about your medical history, your family and social history, and other matters related to your pregnancy. The practitioner will discuss any general health concerns you may have and outline how you will be cared for during your pregnancy. You will have a variety of blood and urine tests (for information on specific tests, see pages 94 to 102). These will give your practitioner an idea of what is normal for you and what aspects of your health may need to be followed closely during your pregnancy. You will have a general physical exam and a pelvic exam. The pelvic exam and a blood test may confirm the pregnancy.

During the pelvic exam, the practitioner will do a Pap smear, if needed, and will assess the size, shape, and structure of your pelvic bones. It's important to remember that your overall body size doesn't necessarily correlate with the size of your pelvic opening. Small women's pelvises are usually wide enough to deliver larger babies. The size of your pelvic opening can't be judged from your external appearance.

> ### Tori's Tip: Note Baby-Related Thoughts in One Spot
>
> Keep a small pad of paper in your purse to use only for questions to ask your practitioner, things to purchase for the baby, ideas for baby names, and other baby-related notes.

Your practitioner will probably prescribe a daily prenatal multivitamin for you. If the level of iron in your blood is low, you might also be prescribed an iron tablet.

You will probably see your practitioner once a month until you are seven months (28 weeks) pregnant. From weeks 29 through 36, you will visit every two weeks, and after week 36, you will see your practitioner once a week.

Diet and Dietary Supplements

Advice about what and how much to eat in pregnancy can be confusing. Here are some simple guidelines for you.

Gaining weight is essential to meeting the nutritional requirements of both you and your baby. Most women need to gain 25 to 30 pounds over the course of a pregnancy. If you are expecting multiples, you will probably gain 35 to 50 pounds or more. Your weight gain will depend partly on whether you are beginning your pregnancy at your ideal weight or are either under- or overweight.

You will want to meet your increased caloric needs primarily by eating healthful foods. It is best to eat fresh fruits and vegetables every day, along with some high-protein foods (meat, poultry, fish, tofu, beans, eggs, nuts) and whole grains such as wheat, oats, and rice.

Calcium-rich foods are necessary for good nutrition, too. If you drink milk, four glasses per day will be enough. You can substitute cheese, yogurt, or other milk products if you wish. If you don't like or cannot tolerate milk products, you'll need to eat other calcium-rich foods, such as tofu, soymilk, broccoli and other greens, nuts, and beans, or take calcium tablets. Canned fish like sardines and salmon contain small, edible bones and are another excellent source of calcium. And don't overdo it with soft drinks. The phosphorus in these drinks raises your blood phosphorus levels, which can result in calcium loss from your bones. Please talk with your practitioner if you're not sure that you are getting enough calcium.

Pregnancy and breastfeeding also require extra iron. As your blood volume increases, the proportion of red blood cells in your circulatory system may decrease. It is important to increase your daily intake of iron-rich foods, such as black beans, lentils, most meats (especially liver), eggs, dandelion leaves, blackstrap molasses, and seaweeds (e.g., nori and arame, available at health-food stores and other specialty food shops and prepared in various ways).

To keep your bowel movements soft, drink six to eight daily glasses of water or other liquids (juice and electrolyte drinks are fine in moderation), and eat plenty of foods high in fiber, such as fruits, vegetables (especially peas and beans), and whole grains. You can easily find commercial breads and cereals that contain bran.

Pregnant women often feel better if they snack throughout the day instead of eating two or three big meals. For this reason, I suggest that you try to balance your nutrients over the course of a day instead of meal by meal.

These are the most common nutrition questions that I hear from moms at this stage of pregnancy:

Q: *How important are my personal eating habits during my pregnancy?*

A: Eating properly is one of the best things you can do for yourself and your growing baby. If you can, eat a wide variety of foods. This can be hard during the first trimester if you are experiencing morning sickness. But try to eat very well in the second and third trimesters. If you tend to eat a lot of sweets or other junk food, now is a good time to decrease those foods in your diet. Processed, high-fat foods and sweets provide "empty" calories and can cause you to gain weight that you don't need (fatty foods such as avocados, nuts, and olive oil, all good sources of vitamin E, are not empty-calorie foods).

Q: *What are the recommended numbers of food servings for a pregnant woman?*

A: The American College of Obstetricians and Gynecologists (ACOG) recommends that pregnant women eat the following amounts daily:

- Nine servings of bread, cereal, rice, or pasta
- Four servings of vegetables
- Three servings of fruits
- Three servings of milk, yogurt, or cheese (I recommend four)
- Three servings of meat, poultry, fish, dry beans, eggs, or nuts
- This may seem like a lot of food, but the servings that ACOG has in mind are small (see box page 80). Between your meals and snacks, you may already be meeting the guidelines.

Q: *Since I am now eating for two, should I be eating a great deal more?*

A: Although you are eating for two, one of you is very small. Many women are hungrier during pregnancy. It's fine to increase the amount you eat to match your appetite, but keep your nutrition balanced, and again, stay clear of empty-calorie foods.

Q: *Must I control my salt intake during pregnancy?*

A: Pregnant women generally don't need to alter the amount of salt in their diet. On the other hand, many of us already use more salt than we need. Manage your salt intake by staying away from high-salt foods, such as chips and most commercially canned foods. Also, don't add much salt as you cook, and keep the shaker off the table. Once you take away the salt, you may enjoy the true taste of your food more.

Q: *Why do I experience bizarre food cravings now that I'm pregnant?*

A: Food cravings during pregnancy are thought to signal a woman's need for extra nutrients. A craving for ice cream, for example, may be

How Much Is a Serving?

When you're checking your diet against ACOG recommendations, you can use this visual guide to estimating serving size:

One serving of bread = one thin slice

One serving of rice = a cupcake wrapper

One serving of potato = a computer mouse

One serving of whole fruit = a tennis ball

One serving of cut fruit = seven cotton balls

One serving of cheese = two 9-volt batteries

One serving of broccoli = a standard light bulb

One serving of fish = a checkbook

One serving of meat = a deck of cards

your body's way of suggesting that you need additional fat or calcium in your diet, not necessarily a pint of vanilla fudge! Many women crave meat for its extra protein; some crave salad or a particular vegetable. Honor your cravings, but be careful not to let the ones for high-fat foods or sweets get out of hand.

VITAMINS

It is best to get vitamins directly from the food you eat. If you maintain a well-balanced and nutritious diet that includes the four food groups (fruits and vegetables, grains, protein foods, and milk products), you shouldn't need supplemental vitamins or minerals. For people who can't always eat well, though, supplements can fill in for what is missing from the diet. Most of us in the United States fail to meet all our nutritional needs from our diet alone, and this is especially true for pregnant women. For this reason, most practitioners prescribe a daily multivitamin specifically designed for the needs of pregnancy, with at least 400 micrograms of folic acid. Take one pill daily, with your largest meal. Multi-vitamins can cause upset stomach and constipation, but these side effects are less likely to occur if you take the pill with your largest daily meal.

Prenatal multivitamins contain minerals, including iron. If your hemoglobin level tests low, however, your practitioner may prescribe a daily iron tablet in addition to a multivitamin. Iron tablets can also cause stomach upset and constipation, so it is important to take them with food. The tablets can also make your stools very dark, because of the excess iron that does not get absorbed in your intestines. This is nothing to worry about.

Medications During Pregnancy

Although it is generally best to avoid medications during your pregnancy, many medications can be safely taken when needed. The most common of these are listed here. *Before taking these or any other medications in pregnancy, always discuss them with your practitioner.*

If you are taking medication for a medical condition when you get pregnant, you may need to continue the medication throughout your pregnancy, or you may be advised to switch to a medication that is safer during pregnancy. It is important to discuss your medications as soon as possible with your practitioner.

Antibiotics. Penicillin, ampicillin, amoxicillin, Keflex, erythromycin, and Zithromax may be safely taken during pregnancy. Avoid tetracycline, sulfa drugs, and quinolones (e.g., Cipro).

Tori's Tip: Choose When to Share the News

Month two is when many couples share the news of the pregnancy with family and friends. If you're ready to do so, enjoy this special, happy time! If you are concerned about the possibility of miscarrying, though, you may be more comfortable waiting a few more weeks. Trust your own instincts in deciding when the time is right.

Aspirin. Although small amounts of aspirin are considered safe until the seventh month of pregnancy, many practitioners prefer that women take acetaminophen (such as Tylenol) for pain relief at any time during pregnancy. To treat some conditions associated with infertility, your doctor may prescribe low-dose aspirin, or baby aspirin, for the first trimester.

Acetaminophen. This mild pain reliever, which you may know by the brand name Tylenol, is safe throughout pregnancy.

Nonsteroidal anti-inflammatory drugs (NSAIDs). Ibuprofen, such as Advil or Motrin, and other NSAIDs are not safe to take during pregnancy. They can promote bleeding, and some studies show they cause an increased rate of miscarriage, although other studies show contradictory results. A bigger concern involves the use of NSAID drugs in the third trimester, when they can cause a heart defect in the baby: a premature closure of the blood vessel known as the ductus arteriosus. This premature closure can cause pulmonary hypertension, or high blood pressure, in the baby's lungs.

Antacids. Calcium carbonate (Tums), aluminum hydroxide magnesium (Maalox, Mylanta, Gelusil), oral magaldrate (Riopan), and milk of magnesia are considered safe throughout pregnancy when taken in moderation and in accordance with a practitioner's advice. Calcium carbonate can also be a source of supplemental calcium.

Antihistamines and cold remedies. There is much debate over whether these medications are harmful to a developing fetus. It is best to avoid the use of any of these drugs during the first 12 weeks of pregnancy. After 12 weeks, pseudoephedrine (Sudafed) and chlorpheniramine (Chlor-trimeton) are considered safe.

Cough medication. Dextromethorphan (Robitussin, Delsym) and guaifenesin (with or without codeine) are considered safe for use in pregnancy, especially after the first 12 weeks.

Opioid pain relievers. Codeine, propoxyphene (Darvon), and hydrocodone (Norco) are considered safe when prescribed by a physician for migraines or other moderate to severe pain unrelieved by acetaminophen.

Local anesthetics. Lidocaine-type drugs, when appropriately used for dental work or other procedures that call for local anesthesia, are considered safe throughout pregnancy.

Surgical anesthetics. These are considered safe when used for emergency and other necessary medical procedures.

Ask Tori, R.N.

HEARING THE BABY'S HEARTBEAT

Hi, Tori,

How many weeks along will I be when my doctor can hear my baby's heartbeat?

—Amber, North Dakota

Dear Amber,

Many physicians now have ultrasound scanners in their offices. With these machines, it is usually possible to see the baby's heart beating at 6 to 8 weeks. Most ultrasound scanners have amplifiers, so you can hear as well as see the heartbeat by this early date. If your doctor or midwife doesn't have an ultrasound scanner, he or she will listen with a Doppler, a small, ultrasonic device that amplifies the sound of the baby's heartbeat. With a Doppler, it's sometimes possible to hear the baby's heartbeat at 6 to 8 weeks, but it's much easier to do so at 11 or 12 weeks.

PHYSICIAN OR MIDWIFE?

Hi, Tori,

A friend of mine told me that I should check into having a midwife at my baby's birth, I don't really understand what they do, Are they better than doctors? Can you explain?

—Melanie, Utah

Dear Melanie,

Midwives care for healthy women who have low-risk pregnancies and uncomplicated deliveries. The philosophy of midwifery is to encourage as natural a labor as possible and to provide continuous support for the laboring woman. Besides typically being present for a longer period during labor than a physician would be, midwives favor low medical intervention. In the hospital, however, they support a women's choice to have epidural anesthesia, and they use other interventions or bring in an obstetrician when necessary.

Certified nurse-midwives (CNMs) frequently share a practice with one or more physicians and consult with them as needed. Having your care provided by a CNM may be more affordable than using a physician. Whether a midwife would be better for you, though, may depend on the level of care you need. In many countries, midwives manage most normal births and leave cesarean or complicated births to their physician colleagues.

Whether to use a physician or midwife is a personal decision. I encourage you to make the choice that feels right for you.

CHEMICALS IN THE WORKPLACE

Dear Tori,

My partner, who is about nine weeks pregnant, does research in environmental chemistry in a laboratory at her university. I am concerned about the chemicals she is in contact with every day. What chemicals might be harmful to our baby, and what precautions should she take if she is working with these chemicals?

—Robert, South Carolina

Dear Robert,

Your partner's employer should have a list of all the chemicals that are used in the workplace. Those that are dangerous to pregnant or lactating women should be posted, and she should not have contact with them. If you have any questions about this, you can contact the Occupational Safety and Health Administration (OSHA), 200 Constitution Avenue NW, Washington, DC 20210. The OSHA website, www.osha.gov, is also an excellent source of information.

COLD MEDICINE

Tori,

I'm 14 weeks pregnant, and I have a bad cold. Can I take any type of over-the-counter antihistamine or decongestant to stop my nose from running? Please help-it's driving me crazy!

−Kristin, Oklahoma

Dear Kristin,

Getting sick while you are pregnant isn't fair! Colds can be especially bothersome if your sinuses are already feeling stuffy from the extra blood flow you now have.

You mentioned both antihistamines and decongestants. Let me differentiate them. An antihistamine relieves the itchy, watery eyes, sneezing, and other symptoms of environmental allergies such as hay fever. Diphenhydramine (Benadryl) is an example of an antihistamine. A decongestant relieves the stuffy nose and ear congestion frequently caused by a common-cold virus or sinus inflammation (sinusitis). A typical decongestant is pseudoephedrine, which comes under a variety of brand names.

Pseudoephedrine is considered safe for use during pregnancy. Until recently, this drug was readily available on grocery and drugstore shelves. Currently, pseudoephedrine products are kept out of reach of shoppers and available only on request. This is because pseudoephedrine is used in the illegal manufacturing of methamphetamine. Although no prescription is necessary in most states, you will have to show your driver's license or other personal identification to buy the drug.

Some cold medication manufacturers have replaced pseudoephedrine with phenylephrine, but many people feel that the replacement does not work as well. Nor has the use of phenylephrine during pregnancy been as well studied as that of pseudoephedrine.

Please talk to your doctor or midwife before taking any of these medications. If you are having aches or a fever, your practitioner may suggest that you take acetaminophen instead. In any case, you should rest as much as possible.

OMEGA-3 FATTY ACIDS

Hi, Tori,

I am ten weeks pregnant with my first baby, and I am kind of a health and vitamin nut. I really believe in omega-3 fatty acids, and I want to continue taking my supplements throughout my pregnancy. What do you think?

—Nicole, Kentucky

Dear Nicole,

Omega-3 fatty acids, docosahexaenoic acid (DHA) and eicosa-pentaenoic acid (EPA), are essential nutrients for optimal fetal and infant neurodevelopment. A recent study has shown that deficiencies of these in pregnancy increase the baby's risk of developmental delays in communication, fine motor, and social skills.

The richest sources of omega-3 fatty acids are oily fish. As discussed on page 43, however, many fish rich in these fatty acids also contain dangerous pollutants such as mercury, a neurotoxin. There is much controversy over how much fish women can safely eat during pregnancy without exposing their babies to too much neurotoxin.

Omega-3 fatty acids are found in pumpkin and flax seeds, but in much lower levels than in oily fish. High-quality omega-3 supplements may be a good alternative. Discuss these with you practitioner.

DAD'S CORNER

Cravings. There are a lot of silly jokes on this subject, but many women really do have cravings in pregnancy—even for Mexican food at two in the morning!

At this time, your partner's body is undergoing intense physiological changes. Everything is altered, including the rate at which she burns calories and the types and combinations of proteins, carbohydrates, vitamins, and minerals that she needs. In essence, your partner's body has become a cauldron for a chemical soup made from a very specific recipe for producing a healthy baby. If your partner craves meat, her body may need protein.

Some cravings are harder to understand. Oddly enough, chewing large amounts of ice can be a sign of anemia. Some women even crave nonfoods such as clay or paint. Such cravings are often caused by nutritional deficiencies and should be addressed by the mother's practitioner.

Nutrition. Matters of diet are best handled as a team. Sit down with your partner, and discuss how you need to adapt the household eating habits for pregnancy. If both of you are very busy, you may find yourself substituting the quick fix of sweets, caffeine, and fast food for wholesome, balanced meals, the best source for baby-building nutrients. If one person is shopping and cooking for the entire household, it will be easier for your partner to eat well if you and everyone else in the household agree to eat healthy foods.

If your partner has morning sickness, this may be a difficult time for her to think about food at all. If she usually does the shopping and cooking, you may need to take over these tasks for a while. Don't worry, though; your partner probably won't want gourmet meals. She may most appreciate familiar "comfort foods" such as grilled cheese sandwiches, cottage cheese, and yogurt. Fruit salads and fresh-cut vegetables can be very refreshing. Try to avoid greasy or spicy foods and certainly anything that is very strong smelling.

As pregnancy progresses, both of you will want to pay extra attention to your eating habits. Poor nutrition can cause abnormal hormonal and blood-sugar levels, which in turn can affect emotions, sleep patterns, physical strength and endurance, and self-esteem. A sound diet maintains a healthy body, helps the baby grow properly, and makes it easier to tell true medical problems from minor upsets. Give your family the gift of good food!

Treat Her Well. This month, you might arrange a lunch for your partner and several of her good friends, so that she can share her happiness (and all her other feelings) with them. One of her friends might help you make up a list and get the group together.

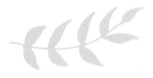

Turning the Corner
YOUR THIRD MONTH: WEEKS 12 THROUGH 15

THE THIRD MONTH IS, I hope, your final month in the Nausea Club, an exclusive organization for expectant mothers. Unlike most clubs, it's one whose members can't wait to leave.

WHAT'S HAPPENING WITH YOUR BABY?

Your baby is continuing to grow very quickly during this time. Her internal organs are almost fully formed, and by the end of this month, she will weigh ½ to 1 ounce (14 to 28 g) and measure 3 to 4 inches (7.6 to 10 cm) long, about the width of the palm of your hand. Her head is growing rapidly, and her face looks like a baby's. She is starting to develop tooth buds, and her fingers and toes are distinct. She even has soft fingernails! Her circulatory system is functioning well, and she is starting to produce small amounts of a saline-like urine called amniotic fluid. This fluid will keep her safely cushioned inside your uterus, in her amniotic sac (which is also called the water bag, bag of waters, amniotic bag, or membrane). Your baby's reproductive organs have formed, but her genitalia are not yet distinct. She is stretching and kicking her tiny legs and moving her entire body. If your practitioner has a Doppler listening device, you may soon be able to hear her heartbeat. Don't worry, though, if you can't. You will be able to hear it in a few weeks.

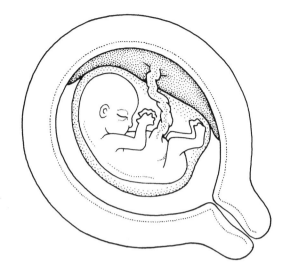

WHAT'S HAPPENING WITH YOUR BODY?

As you move into your second trimester, pregnancy may begin to feel different. In the early weeks, you may have experienced nausea, great fatigue, disbelief at being pregnant, and even some ambivalence about the pregnancy. Now that your estrogen levels are rising and your progesterone levels are falling, you are probably feeling less nauseated and your appetite is probably returning, maybe with intensity. You may still sleep a lot, but you probably feel an increase in energy. Under the influence of estrogen, sometimes called "the happy hormone," many women experience a new sense of calmness and joy about their pregnancies in the second trimester. This may be when you first share your news and enjoy the support and excitement of others.

At this time, too, you are beginning to see and feel your expanding uterus. You can feel the smooth bulge appearing above your pubic bone, and you realize that your shape is truly changing.

You may also be experiencing mood changes similar to those you may have had during your menstrual cycle. You may feel happy and

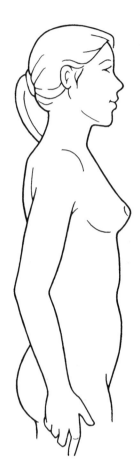

elated at times and irritable, weepy, or overwhelmed at others. You may sometimes feel scattered and forgetful. Mood changes can strike with no warning, and they can be alarming. You may need to ask for some extra TLC from your partner during these times.

IMPORTANT THINGS TO KNOW

While you are attending to your own and your growing baby's physical health, it is also important to begin planning how your pregnancy will affect your work. The following pages offer information on both the health and career aspects of having a baby.

Is There Such a Thing as "Pregnancy Brain"?

Women sometimes humorously use this term for the forgetfulness that seems to appear during pregnancy (the same condition is called "mommy brain" after the baby is born). Is this condition real?

Studies show that hormonal changes do affect memory function, and fatigue affects both memory and the ability to process thoughts. Besides, a pregnant woman has a lot on her mind—the baby, a changing relationship with her partner, work and financial concerns, and more. All these things can make you feel a little scatterbrained.

Rest, even a short catnap, can refresh you and sharpen your mind. And take heart: Some recent research has shown that motherhood ultimately increases a woman's intelligence.

Your Prenatal Checkup

This month's visit will be quite typical of your regular checkups. During this appointment, your doctor or midwife will check the growth of your baby by assessing the growth of your uterus. The practitioner will place one hand on your lower abdomen at your pubic bone and, with the other, feel for the top of the uterus, or the *fundus*. At this stage, your fundus will be midway between your pubic bone and your navel. Your practitioner will assess the baby's growth at each subsequent visit by checking where your fundus is.

At this visit, it will be easy to hear the baby's heartbeat with the Doppler device. Your practitioner will ask you if you have felt the baby move yet. You may or may not have. If not, don't worry; you will very soon.

You will be weighed. You will probably have gained about 6 to 8 pounds (2.7 to 3.6 kg) by now. If your weight gain is of concern, your practitioner will talk with you about it.

You will have a blood-pressure check, too. The reading will serve as your baseline, or norm, for your pregnancy. During pregnancy, a woman's blood pressure is normally about the same as or a bit lower

Twins' Moms Feel and Look More Pregnant

Moms carrying more than one baby typically have higher levels of pregnancy hormones in their bodies, which can lead to more pronounced pregnancy symptoms, such as fatigue, nausea, and hunger.

Discovering that you are expecting twins can be emotionally and physically overwhelming. It is common for a twins' mom's emotions to alternate between happy excitement and apprehension.

Mothers of twins can also expect to become larger than a woman carrying one baby, and to "show" much sooner. A twins' mom's uterus is approximately 6 to 8 weeks larger than that of a mom with one baby. So ... at 24 weeks' gestation with twins, you may look like you are 32 weeks along! Many women who are pregnant with twins start showing by the end of their first trimester.

than before pregnancy. If it is higher, your doctor will watch it closely throughout your pregnancy.

Hypertension is the most common medical problem during pregnancy, affecting 2 to 3 percent of pregnancies. There are three hypertensive disorders of pregnancy: *chronic hypertension, gestational hypertension*, and *preeclampsia*. Chronic hypertension begins before pregnancy; gestational hypertension begins during the latter half of pregnancy. Preeclampsia is a poorly understood disease of the third trimester; if left untreated, the disease can endanger both mother and baby. I'll discuss preeclampsia more later (see page 194).

A sample of your urine will be checked for both sugar (glucose) and protein at this visit and all subsequent ones. You should normally have neither sugar nor protein in your urine, although if they appear just once, this may be nothing to worry about.

You will have time to ask questions or to talk about your concerns. If you think of questions between visits, it may help to keep a list to bring with you so that you don't forget what you wanted to discuss.

Fetal Testing

An assortment of prenatal tests is available to identify physical defects in the fetus, chromosomal abnormalities such as Down syndrome, and genetic anomalies such as sickle-cell anemia. There are two general types of fetal tests: screening and diagnostic. Screening tests, including ultrasound and maternal blood tests, provide the information needed to determine whether diagnostic testing should be conducted. Diagnostic tests definitively show the absence or presence of a fetal abnormality.

In the past, fetal diagnostic tests were primarily offered to women who were over 35 or who had a family history of a genetic problem. Recently, however, the American College of Obstetricians and Gynecologists (ACOG) issued a recommendation that all women, regardless of age or family history, be offered fetal diagnostic testing.

Your choice of tests should be based on what you will do with the information. You'll want to discuss with your practitioner the risks and benefits of each proposed test. Women frequently tell me that testing has provided them with the information they needed to make the best decisions possible for themselves.

Here are some things to consider when deciding whether to have fetal testing:

- What will you do with the test results? Normal results can ease your mind. But if a test indicates that your baby may have a birth defect, you may be faced with a difficult decision. Will you choose to terminate your pregnancy? Or will you use the knowledge to prepare yourself for caring for a challenged child?

- How will you handle a false test result? Fetal tests aren't perfect. The frequency of inaccurate results varies from test to test.

- What are the risks? Some tests can cause anxiety, pain, or, rarely, miscarriage. Weigh these risks against the value of knowing the results.

If you will be having your baby in a smaller community hospital or birth center, the facility might not offer testing. Your practitioner may have you go to a larger city or to a teaching hospital for a test.

The following sections describe the most common types of fetal tests and why and how they are done. Some of them are done during the first trimester and some in the second, but I'll outline them all here.

STANDARD TESTING

1.) Ultrasound

You may have had this test already. It can be performed anytime in pregnancy, by a woman's practitioner or by a specially trained technician, for a variety of reasons. Ultrasound has not been shown to cause any harm to mother or baby.

Ultrasound is most commonly used

- to confirm a baby's gestational age,
- to identify the location of the pregnancy (to rule out an ectopic pregnancy),
- to study the placenta and investigate any bleeding problems,
- to identify a multiple pregnancy,
- to identify possible fetal abnormalities,
- to assist with another prenatal test (to guide the needle with amniocentesis or chorionic villus sampling), or
- to assess the growth, position, and well-being of the baby.

In today's obstetrical practices, many women have two or more ultrasound scans. The first is done early in the pregnancy, to confirm the baby's gestational age, and the second is done at approximately 18 to 22 weeks. The second-trimester scan is used to assess the baby's size and look for abnormalities. This ultrasound is referred to as a Fetal Survey. Additional ultrasounds will be performed based on the medical need.

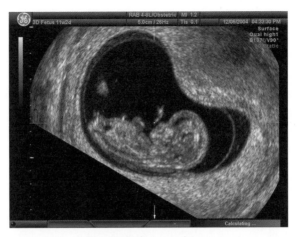

Standard Ultrasound Scan

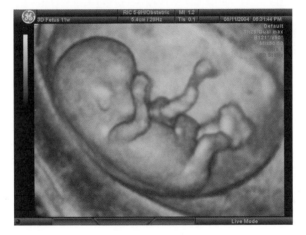

3-D Ultrasound Scan

An ultrasound scan is performed either on your abdomen (*abdominal ultrasound*) or inside your vagina (*transvaginal ultrasound*). The scan is painless to you and your baby. The ultrasound transducer transmits high-frequency sound waves that travel through the amniotic fluid and bounce off the curves and variations in your body, including your baby. These sound waves are then translated into visible dark and light areas to create an image of your baby, a *sonogram*, on a monitor screen and on film.

A *standard* ultrasound scan, which takes 15 to 20 minutes, creates a two-dimensional image. An *advanced or high-definition* ultrasound uses more sophisticated equipment and can be targeted to check suspected problems; this is the scan typically done during the second trimester. The newest type of ultrasound provides three-dimensional (3-D) images, often with photo-quality detail. In my medical center, 3-D ultrasound is used by perinatologists to check on possible problems identified by advanced ultrasounds.

2.) Glucose Intolerance Screening & Anemia

Between 24 to 28 weeks, a Glucose Load Test is recommended for all pregnant women for each pregnancy. This test involves drinking a sugar-filled liquid and having your blood drawn one hour after consumption to see how efficiently your body is processing sugar. During this blood draw, you are also likely to be tested for low hemoglobin or anemia.

3.) The Rh Factor

Your blood will be tested for the Rh factor. Rh disease is a pregnancy complication in which your immune system attacks the baby's blood and can result in a life-threatening situation for the baby if left untreated. Fortunately, it can be prevented with a shot called Rhogam, which is given at 28 weeks or anytime a vaginal bleed occurs. If your blood type is negative, then you may be at risk for Rh disease, which affects about 10 percent of people.

OPTIONAL TESTING
Screening Tests
1.) INTEGRATED SCREENING

This is a combination of two blood samples drawn in the first and second trimesters (AFP Quadruple Marker) combined with a nuchal translucency measurement (ultrasound) at around 12 weeks.

2.) QUAD SCREEN TESTING

This screening blood test, also known as the multiple marker test, is performed between the 15th and 18th weeks of pregnancy. The test measures the levels of four substances:

- Maternal serum alpha-fetoprotein (MAFP), a protein produced by the fetus
- Human chorionic gonadotropin (hCG), a hormone produced by the placenta
- Estriol, a form of estrogen produced by both the placenta and the fetus
- Inhibin-A, a protein produced by the placenta and ovaries

Particularly high or low levels of these substances can be a sign of an abnormality in the baby. High levels of MAFP may suggest that the fetus has a neural-tube defect such as spina bifida, which causes a deformity of the brain or spinal cord. Low levels of MAFP and abnormal levels of hCG and estriol may indicate trisomy 21 (Down syndrome) or trisomy 18 (Edwards syndrome). The results are considered along with the mother's age and ethnic background to estimate the probability of these and other genetic disorders.

False positive results are common with quad screen testing. Approximately 6 percent of women who take the test get a positive result, and only a very small fraction of these will have a baby with a defect. The accuracy of the test depends partly on timing. The majority of false positive results occur either because the pregnancy is further along, or less so, than the mother and her practitioner thought or because the mother is pregnant with twins, triplets, or more.

If your first test results are even slightly abnormal, the test will be repeated. If your second results are also abnormal, your doctor will recommend that you have an advanced, high-definition ultrasound scan, amniocentesis, or both. The quad screen test cannot diagnose a birth defect; it just indicates that more testing is needed.

What Is Trisomy?

Humans normally have 23 pairs of chromosomes in each cell. Each pair of chromosomes holds a particular position in the cell and carries certain genetic material. A trisomy occurs when a baby has three chromosomes, instead of the normal two, in one position.

The most common three-chromosome arrangement is trisomy 21, also known as Down syndrome. A baby with Down syndrome has three of the twenty-first chromosome. This extra chromosome causes a combination of physical and mental abnormalities. In 2006, the Centers for Disease Control and Prevention (CDC) estimated that 1 in every 733 births in the United States was a baby with trisomy 21. The risk of conceiving a baby with Down syndrome rises with the mother's age. At age 22, the risk is 1 in 1,490; at age 40, it is 1 in 60.

Trisomy 18, or Edward syndrome, occurs when a baby has three of the 18th chromosome. Trisomy 18 occurs in 1 of about 3,000 births. Unlike Down syndrome, trisomy 18 is usually fatal. Most babies with this syndrome die before birth or soon thereafter.

Even though quad screen testing can make you anxious, it is still a valuable screening tool. As with so many things, understanding the facts surrounding an issue can lessen your anxiety. Most importantly, remember that diagnostic tests following positive quad screen tests usually show that a baby does not have Down syndrome, trisomy 18, or a neural-tube defect. In approximately 97 percent of abnormal quad screen test results, the baby turns out to be normal.

3.) FIRST-TRIMESTER ULTRA-SCREEN

This noninvasive screening test combines a maternal blood analysis with a specialized ultrasound exam to identify the likelihood of specific chromosomal abnormalities, including Down syndrome (the test does not screen for neural-tube defects). Performed between 11 and 13 weeks of pregnancy, Ultra-Screen is currently considered the most accurate noninvasive method available for screening for chromosomal abnormalities. Its accuracy rate in detecting chromosomal abnormalities is approximately 85 percent.

The Ultra-Screen blood analysis measures the levels of the pregnancy hormones hCG and PAPP-A (pregnancy-associated plasma protein A). Abnormally high or low levels of these are often found in babies with chromosomal abnormalities.

The ultrasound portion of the test measures the *nuchal translucency*, or the thickness of the tissue at the back of the baby's neck. Babies with chromosomal abnormalities tend to accumulate more fluid at the back of the neck during the first trimester than do other babies, and the collected fluid causes the tissue to be thicker and therefore less translucent. Through thousands of screenings, researchers have determined a normal range of nuchal thickness.

The results of the two parts of the test are considered along with the mother's age to determine whether a baby is likely to have a chromosomal abnormality. As with quad screen testing, positive results signal the need for more testing. False positive results occur at a rate of 5 percent.

Diagnostic Tests

1.) CHORIONIC VILLUS SAMPLING

Chorionic villus sampling (CVS) is a diagnostic test to detect fetal abnormalities. It may be chosen over amniocentesis because it can be done earlier in the pregnancy, between 10 and 13 weeks from the first day of the last menstrual period. The major defects that can be detected are Down syndrome, Tay-Sachs (see page 112), thalassemia major and minor (page 112), sickle-cell anemia (page 112), and cystic fibrosis (page 103).

The CVS procedure is performed in a perinatal medical center or hospital, by either a perinatologist or a geneticist-physician. A sample is taken through the mother's abdomen or, more commonly, through the vagina and cervix. With the help of ultrasound, a very thin tube is inserted into the uterus, and a tiny tissue sample of the chorionic villi is taken from outside the sac where the baby develops. The chorionic villi are the fingerlike projections of the chorion, which is the membrane that will become the fetal side of the placenta. Results are often available within a week.

The level of physical discomfort experienced with CVS varies from woman to woman, but many women feel emotionally exhausted after the procedure, and some have spotting or mild cramping afterward. In less than 1 percent of cases, CVS causes miscarriage. For this reason, it is important to have plenty of emotional support before and after the procedure.

2.) AMNIOCENTESIS

Like CVS, this diagnostic test definitively identifies fetal abnormalities, primarily chromosomal ones such as Down syndrome. If members of your family have had certain birth defects, if you have had a child or a prior pregnancy with a birth defect, or if you have had an abnormal maternal serum alpha-fetoprotein (MAFP) test result, your practitioner may suggest amniocentesis.

Besides identifying genetic abnormalities, amniocentesis can serve in paternity testing. DNA obtained from the baby during amniocentesis is compared with DNA collected from the possible father. The results are 99 percent accurate.

Amniocentesis is typically done between weeks 16 and 18 of pregnancy, although it is done earlier or later in certain cases. Some medical centers can perform amniocentesis as early as 11 weeks. Practitioners sometimes use the procedure late in pregnancy if the baby might be born early, to assess whether his lungs are mature enough for him to breathe on his own.

Amniocentesis may be performed in a prenatal testing center or in a physician's office. Amniotic fluid contains cells shed by the fetus. A long, thin, hollow needle is inserted through the mother's abdomen and into the uterus. Guided by ultrasound, the doctor withdraws a small amount of amniotic fluid and sends it to a laboratory, where cells shed by the fetus and contained in the fluid are analyzed. Getting results can take from a few days to two weeks. Amniocentesis will definitely reveal the baby's gender, so be sure you and your partner have talked about whether or not you would like to know.

Some women feel cramping or pressure during the procedure, but others say it doesn't hurt at all. Occasionally, cramping, spotting, or a little leakage of amniotic fluid occurs for a short time afterward. Most physicians recommend that you take it easy for the rest of the day after your amniocentesis.

Miscarriage can result after amniocentesis if the procedure causes tearing of the amniotic sac or an infection in the uterus. The risk of miscarriage, however, is only 0.5 percent, or 1 in 200.

Vaccinations

The Centers for Disease Control (CDC) recommends that women pregnant during flu season receive the flu shot. Also, pregnant women who haven't had a dose of Tdap (a vaccine to protect mom and baby against tetanus, diphtheria, and pertussis) should get one after 20 weeks. Receiving the vaccine in pregnancy gives your baby extra protection against whooping cough, which can be very dangerous for newborns.

Carrier Testing for Cystic Fibrosis

Cystic fibrosis is a genetic condition that causes the body to produce extreme amounts of abnormally thick, sticky mucus. The mucus collects primarily in the lungs, which causes severe respiratory problems and frequent episodes of pneumonia. It can also affect the internal organs, resulting in intestinal and growth difficulties.

It is an inherited recessive condition, which means that a child can only have the disease if both parents carry the specific abnormal gene. If both parents are carriers, there is a 25 percent chance that their baby with have cystic fibrosis. If only one parent carries the mutated gene, the child will not develop the disease. However, the gene can be passed on to the child, making him or her a carrier. Because there are no symptoms and most people do not even know they have the gene.

Cystic fibrosis is most common in Caucasians and least common in Asian Americans. A person can learn if he or she is a carrier with a blood test looking for DNA mutations. More specific testing through an amniocenteses or CVS (chorionic villi sampling) will determine if the baby has the actual disease. There have been many improvements in treatment options, but today there is no cure.

What Is a High-Risk Pregnancy?

The term *high-risk* is applied to a pregnancy when the mother or baby needs specialized monitoring. Yours might be considered a high-risk pregnancy if any of the following conditions apply:

- You are carrying more than one baby.
- You are older (than 40, usually).
- You have a medical condition such as epilepsy, high blood pressure, lupus, or insulin-dependent diabetes.
- You have had preterm labor in a prior pregnancy.

Any of these situations increases your risk for complications during pregnancy, birth, or both.

A woman with a high-risk pregnancy is usually cared for by a regular obstetrician-gynecologist. If needed, the OB-GYN refers a woman to a perinatologist, an obstetrician who is specially trained to manage high-risk pregnancies.

Pregnancy and Maternity Leave

If you have not already alerted your employer to your pregnancy, you will want to tell your direct supervisor—and the human resources department, if there is one—before your pregnancy becomes obvious (this may be sooner than you expected if you are pregnant with multiples). First, though, you should know what your rights are as a pregnant employee:

Disability during pregnancy. If you are temporarily unable to perform your job because of a condition related to your pregnancy, your employer must treat you the same as any other temporarily disabled

What's So Risky About Pregnancy Over 40?

With recent advances in infertility treatments, many women who would have been beyond childbearing age in the past are becoming mothers today. If you are pregnant past forty, you face higher risks of miscarriage (page 51), ectopic pregnancy (page 54), fetal chromosomal abnormalities (page 100), gestational diabetes (page 195), preeclampsia (page 194), placenta previa (page 196), placental abruption (page 306), and cesarean section (page 304). You are also more likely than younger women are to be pregnant with multiples, to go into labor and give birth prematurely, and to have a baby with a low birth weight.

employee—for example, by providing you with an alternative assignment, modified tasks, disability leave, or leave without pay.

Right to work. As a pregnant employee, you have the right to work as long as you are able to perform your job. If you are absent from work because of a pregnancy-related condition, and then you recover, your employer cannot require you to remain on leave until the baby's birth. Nor can your employer prohibit you from returning to work for a predetermined length of time after childbirth.

Right to leave. The U.S. Family Medical Leave Act entitles female and male employees who have worked for an employer for at least 12 months (and at least 1,250 hours) to 12 unpaid workweeks of leave during a 12-month period for (1) a child's birth or placement for adoption or foster care, (2) the serious health condition of a spouse, child, or parent, or (3) the employee's own serious health condition.

Today many U.S. companies and a handful of U.S. states offer *paid* family leave. This is certainly a step forward, but the United States still falls far short of other industrialized nations in support for fami-

What Is the Pregnancy Discrimination Act?

This act is an amendment to Title VII of the Civil Rights Act of 1964. Under the Pregnancy Discrimination Act, an employer cannot discriminate against an employee because of pregnancy, childbirth, or a related medical condition.

lies. Sweden, for example, offers all working parents 18 months of paid leave per child. To encourage the involvement of both parents in child rearing, Swedish law requires each parent to use a minimum of 3 of the 18 months.

Right to job position. As an employee returning from a pregnancy-related absence, you have a right to either the same position you had before your leave or a position equivalent in pay, benefits, and other terms of employment, without any loss of seniority.

Right to health insurance. An employer that provides health insurance must cover any expenses for pregnancy-related conditions in the same manner as for other medical conditions. Additional deductibles can't be imposed for pregnancy-related conditions.

TELLING YOUR BOSS

There is no perfect time to tell your boss about your pregnancy, but you should do it before one of your colleagues does! It is a good idea to plan the time and place for your announcement and to think through what you want to say. Here are some suggestions:

- Select a relatively stress-free time when you and your boss can speak privately without feeling rushed.
- Be sure that you know your rights as an employee before heading into the meeting. This will help you to best respond to your boss's questions.
- Think through the questions your boss may have, and be prepared to talk about his or her concerns. Your boss will probably

want to know how long you plan to be off work, who will replace you when you are gone, how you will help train that person, whether you might not return, and whether there are other ways your pregnancy may affect the company. You may not have definitive answers, of course, and you may not want to share all the answers you have. If you know you won't return to work after the birth, for example, you probably shouldn't tell your boss yet.

- Do not apologize for being pregnant or promise to maintain your full workload throughout the pregnancy. You do not know how you will feel or what may occur as you move through your pregnancy. You are not letting your employer down; you have started (or are adding to) your family.

- Mention that you may occasionally need to leave the office for a prenatal appointment or test.

- Try not to anticipate that your boss will be thrilled about your pregnancy. It will be wonderful if he or she is as happy as you are, but you can't expect this.

FINANCES

Financial matters are a significant source of stress for new parents. The more you plan, the less stressful the changes will be. Sit down with your spouse, and talk through how you will manage your finances over the coming months. Consider the costs of birth and caring for a baby, as

How Much Does Child-Care Cost?

Usually, quite a lot! Costs for full-time infant care in the United States range from $4,000 to $14,000 per year, depending on the region and the type of care (group or one-on-one, in the parents' home, in another family's home, or in a day-care center). To find out about local rates, call a child-care resource and referral agency. You can find one through Child Care Aware (800-424-2246; www.childcareaware.org).

well as the loss of income while you are off work. Don't assume that you will figure all this out after the baby comes. Although you won't want to set any plans in stone before your baby arrives, thinking through all the possibilities now may allow you maximum flexibility later and save you a great deal of stress besides.

You will probably fund part of your maternity leave through short-term disability, if your state or employer offers it, as well as saved vacation days and any personal or sick days you have accumulated. Short-term disability generally covers 6 weeks of leave for birth and the postpartum period; 2 weeks may be added for a cesarean birth or complications. The benefits typically cover from 50 to 60 percent of a person's salary. Under federal law, you can combine your disability leave with as much as 12 weeks of unpaid leave.

How long you work during your pregnancy will depend on many things, including how your pregnancy is going and what type of work you do. Some women, especially those expecting multiples, are advised to stop working, decrease their level of activity, or both, but most continue to work until they feel ready to stop.

Here are some other things to think about:

- Are there any household expenses that you could decrease? What lifestyle changes might help your family get by without your salary for some period of weeks or months?
- Do you want to go back to work after the baby is born? Full-time or part-time?
- Would it be possible for you to be a stay-at-home mom? If so, for how long?
- Could you work at home one or two days a week?
- Would your company consider a proposal for job sharing? This would mean that you would work part-time, splitting your job with someone else.
- Could you consider starting a home-based business?
- If you go back to work full-time or part-time, how much will child-care cost?

Ask Tori, R.N.

RH FACTOR

Dear Tori,

My doctor's nurse phoned this week to ask if I knew that my blood type was Rh-negative. I had been told this years ago but had forgotten about it. The nurse said that if my husband is also Rh-negative (we will find out this week), I have nothing to worry about. If he is not, I have to receive a shot at 28 weeks. Can you please explain why this is necessary?

—Stephanie, Iowa

Dear Stephanie,

Rh factor, or Rh antigen, is a substance present by heredity in the blood of most people. Only 15 percent of us lack Rh factor, or have Rh-negative blood. Years ago, babies often died from what was known as Rh incompatibility, or rhesus disease. Today, we can prevent this from happening.

If both you and your husband have Rh-negative blood, then the baby will also have this blood type, and no treatment is needed. If, however, your blood is Rh-negative and your husband's is Rh-positive, the baby may have Rh-positive blood. In this case, your body could begin producing antibodies to your baby's red blood cells.

If you have never been pregnant before, your baby would be unaffected by these antibodies. They would remain dormant and harmless unless you became pregnant again. Then, if your baby were Rh-positive, the antibodies could cross the placenta and attack the baby's red blood cells. This could cause anemia and mild to severe jaundice in the baby.

To prevent this problem, an Rh-negative mother with an Rh-positive partner receives a shot of Rh immune globulin, or RhoGAM, at 28 weeks of pregnancy and again within 72 hours of giving birth. Rh immune globulin is also given to an Rh-negative woman after a miscarriage, an ectopic pregnancy, or an induced abortion, and at the time of amniocentesis, CVS, or another invasive procedure during pregnancy. A shot of RhoGAM should be considered, too, if an Rh-negative woman experiences any significant bleeding or blunt trauma, such as from a car accident or fall, while she is pregnant. This kind of injury can also cause Rh sensitization.

SLEEPING ON YOUR BACK

Hi, Tori,

I enjoy sleeping on my back, and I have heard that I shouldn't do this. Can you please tell me why, and at what point in pregnancy I should stop?

—Amy, Maine

Amy,

A major blood vessel known as the inferior vena cava runs up your back from your legs. It is responsible for returning blood to your heart. As your uterus and your belly grow, there is increased pressure on this vessel when you are lying flat on your back. You know that you've been in this position too long if you have the sensation that your legs are falling asleep or you just feel uncomfortable. As your pregnancy progresses, you will probably be more comfortable lying on your side. This position allows maximum blood flow through your body and to your placenta and baby.

We all move around a great deal while we are sleeping. Please don't worry if you wake up on your back; this is perfectly normal. Just reposition yourself so that you are comfortable.

GENETIC COUNSELING

Hi, Tori,

I am 39 years old, and my husband and I are undergoing infertility treatment. My doctor has suggested that we see a genetic counselor. Can you tell me a little bit about what genetic counselors do?

—Sarah, Indiana

Dear Sarah,

A genetic counselor is a specially trained health professional who works with a couple to determine their risk of passing on an inheritable disease to their baby. The counselor thoroughly investigates the personal and family health history and ancestry of both mother and father. He or she helps the couple interpret information about a particular disorder, learn about inheritance patterns and the risks that a disease will recur, and review available options.

You might be referred to genetic counseling if any of the following conditions apply:

- You are over 35 years old.
- You have had an abnormal result on a fetal screening test.
- You are planning an invasive, diagnostic fetal test.
- You or the father has already had a child with a birth defect or genetic disorder.
- A close family member has an inherited disease.
- You or the father has any family history of mental retardation, birth defects, or a genetic disease such as muscular dystrophy or cystic fibrosis.
- You and the father are of African, Jewish, Italian, Greek, or Middle Eastern ancestry.

Particular inherited genetic defects, such as the following conditions or diseases, are more likely to occur among people of particular ancestry:

Sickle-cell anemia is found among African Americans. This is a disease in which the body makes abnormally shaped red blood cells.

Tay-Sachs disease occurs in descendants of Central and Eastern European Jews. This is a fatal disorder in which harmful quantities of a fatty substance called *ganglioside* GM2 build up in tissues and nerve cells in the fetal brain.

Thalassemia is a blood disorder that occurs in people of Italian, Greek, Middle Eastern, and Southeast Asian descent. People with the disease are unable to make enough hemoglobin and so become severely anemic.

Genetic counseling is unnecessary for most couples, but it can be very helpful if you fall into one or more of these risk categories.

WHEN WILL I START SHOWING?

Tori,

I am currently 13½ weeks pregnant with my first baby. I am so excited! When can I expect to start showing? My sister is expecting her third baby close to mine, and she is already wearing maternity clothes.

—Keisha, Rhode Island

Keisha,

Different women begin to show at different times. When you will start to show depends on your overall body size, your height, your pre-pregnancy weight, and, especially, the length of your midbody. Women with longer midbodies tend to hide their babies longer and look smaller than do other women whose babies are at the same gestational age. Women who have already given birth, as your sister has, tend to show a little earlier in a subsequent pregnancy. How the baby is positioned in the uterus also partly determines how the mother's body looks.

Most women have at least a little bump by 15 weeks. At first, though, you and your partner may be the only ones to notice your bump. Often, other people don't recognize that a woman is pregnant until she is about 20 weeks along. Although I am petite, when I was pregnant with Alexander, I did not develop even a bump until 16 weeks. I wore maternity clothes because I was excited, but I really didn't need them until I was six months along.

Try not to be concerned about comments such as "Oh, you look so small!" (People may be asking your sister, "Wow! Is that just one baby in there?") No one can tell, just by looking at you, what size your baby is.

PREGNANT AND OVERWEIGHT

Tori,

Although I tried to lose weight before conceiving, I started pregnancy nearly 40 pounds (18 kg) overweight. My doctor has told me that I do not need to gain any weight and that I should just try not to lose any. He has given me suggestions about sensible eating, and I am committed to following them. Besides eating well, I am walking a great deal. I know that much of the weight gained in pregnancy goes to the placenta, baby, extra blood flow, and fluid. How, then, is it possible for overweight women not to gain?

—Jamie, California

Dear Jamie,

It is wonderful that you have a sensible approach to weight and nutrition and that you are doing everything possible to keep yourself and your baby healthy.

Obesity in pregnancy is associated with a higher incidence of hypertension (high blood pressure), preeclampsia, gestational diabetes, and macrosomic babies (heavier than 9½ pounds). Poor eating habits can cause obese women to gain even more weight in pregnancy. But overweight women who eat sensibly often discover that they gain very little during pregnancy. With proper diet and exercise, the body redistributes some of the weight. Some of the existing fat stores are used for the baby, the placenta, and breast tissue. This can happen without extreme dieting. It's important, in fact, not to strictly limit calories during pregnancy and while you are breastfeeding.

If you need help in managing your weight, ask your doctor about visiting with a dietitian or nutritionist. He or she can help you develop a healthy approach to eating and nutritious meal plans.

DAD'S CORNER

At the beginning of the chapter, I mentioned that now, during her third month of pregnancy, the nausea and the extreme fatigue that may have plagued Mom in her first trimester would, hopefully, be passing. She may be starting to show, too, and you and she may have seen your baby in an ultrasound scan. As things change for your partner, you might notice some changes in yourself. You might be feeling pregnant. Seriously!

The Couvade. Many partners of pregnant women undergo a series of symptoms and changes that can mimic some of those typical of

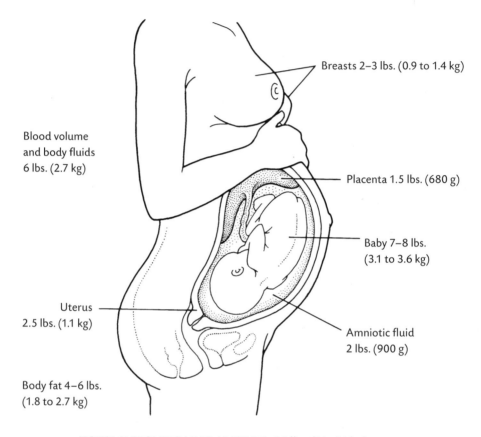

Breasts 2–3 lbs. (0.9 to 1.4 kg)

Blood volume and body fluids 6 lbs. (2.7 kg)

Placenta 1.5 lbs. (680 g)

Baby 7–8 lbs. (3.1 to 3.6 kg)

Uterus 2.5 lbs. (1.1 kg)

Amniotic fluid 2 lbs. (900 g)

Body fat 4–6 lbs. (1.8 to 2.7 kg)

TOTAL WEIGHT GAIN RANGE 25–35 lbs. (11–16 kg)

pregnancy. Most common are mood swings, food cravings, and weight gain. This syndrome, called the couvade, is thought to be experienced by at least 10 percent of partners. It can be a pesky experience, especially for a dad who assumed he was going to observe pregnancy, not share in it.

You can take inspiration from cultures that celebrate the couvade all over the world. In southern India, for example, the experience is ritualized by dressing the husband in women's clothes and laying him in a darkened room while his wife is in labor. This practice is believed to protect the laboring mother and her child by distracting evil forces. When the child is born, the father emerges from his "womb" and rejoins his family. In a way, he is born again, as a father instead of a son.

So, if you are one of those partners who wakes bolt upright in bed with leg cramps, it might help to think, as you rub your calves, that there is probably a father-to-be on the other side of the world doing the same thing.

The Role of Dad in Finances. Common concerns for many expectant couples are careers and finances. A new pregnancy can make one or both partners decide it is time for change. Some people say that they don't want to become a parent while still doing X, Y, or Z. Many dads, in particular, feel a surge of personal growth during pregnancy. They suddenly have the courage to do things they have always dreamed about—buy a house, start a business, go back to school. Often, fathers feel they must find a way to make more money: "If she is going to carry the baby, I should carry the bills."

Analyzing your financial situation is a good idea, but consider carefully before making major changes that may add more stress to your lives. You might augment your savings just by reining in your spending. Money may always be a concern, but what will make any financial stress bearable is the bond you have with your partner. Try not to let worries about the future spoil the wonder and joy of this very special time.

Gardening As Exercise?

Gardening is more than an amusing hobby or a way to get fresh vegetables. Research has shown that it is also good exercise. It can provide a workout that is challenging but less stressful to the body than, say, running or weightlifting (although, as with any other activity, it is important to use proper techniques when you are lifting, bending, or carrying anything in the garden). Gardening is also a relaxing activity, great for providing a mental break and relieving stress. For me, it is a moving meditation.

Treat Her Well. Surprise your partner with a funny pregnancy card, and include a gift certificate or tickets for a comedy show or movie. This is the time to enjoy some of the special things you do as a couple—things that may be harder to manage after the baby is born.

Tori's Tip: Exercise

As you advance into your second trimester, you may feel more energetic than you did a couple of weeks ago. The idea of getting some exercise may sound appealing!

If you were physically active before pregnancy and your doctor or midwife hasn't told you otherwise, you shouldn't have to limit your exercise solely because you are pregnant. Workout activities such as running, bicycling, and weightlifting should be fine. If, however, you participate in a contact sport such as kickboxing or soccer, you should talk with your doctor or midwife before continuing.

If you were not particularly active before pregnancy, I suggest that you begin a flexible regimen of daily walks and stretching or yoga. Yoga or another stretching regimen is a wonderful way to prepare your body, mind, and spirit for mothering. Walking will help your body adjust to your changing center of gravity, which may sometimes make you feel off balance or cause some backache. With walking, it's easy to pace yourself and increase your efforts as you feel ready to do so, and you can enjoy the outdoors at the same time. You might park your car a bit farther away from work, or take a walk at lunchtime. Be sure to wear low-heeled, comfortable shoes.

Even with a gentle workout, be careful not to become overheated. Take rest breaks as needed, and drink plenty of extra water. Remember, you're drinking for two now!

For more exercise tips, see pages 136 and 146 to 153.

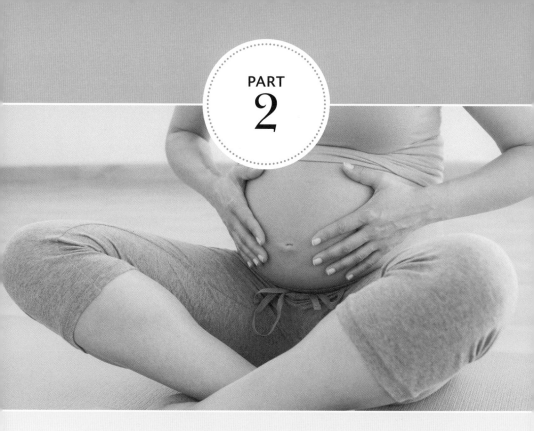

THE SECOND TRIMESTER

Growing and Glowing
YOUR FOURTH MONTH: WEEKS 16 THROUGH 19

AH, FINALLY THE REWARDS FOR THE COMPLETION of the often unnoticed work of the first trimester. In this month, you're likely to find that your energy is back, you feel pregnant, you look pregnant, and, most wonderful of all, you feel your baby move, at last!

WHAT'S HAPPENING WITH YOUR BABY?

During this month, your baby will grow to be 6 to 7 inches long (15 to 18 cm) and ¼ to ½ pound (113 to 227 g) in weight, about as heavy as an orange. His organs are fully developed and functioning well, although if he were born now, he could not live outside your body. His face is really starting to look like a baby's. His eyes are quite large relative to his other facial features. He is also developing the reflexes that will later allow him to suck and swallow. His vocal cords and taste buds have developed, and if you could see him, you might even catch him sucking his thumb! His scalp, hair, eyebrows, and lashes are growing, and his little body is covered with a fine, downy hair called lanugo, which will either disappear before he is born or rub off soon afterward.

Is It a Boy or a Girl?

Given the opportunity to find out, about half of soon-to-be parents choose to do so. The rest wait to be surprised.

Although genetic testing, such as with amniocentesis (page 102) or chorionic villus sampling (page 101), is the only certain way to know your baby's sex before birth, ultrasound is at least 85 percent accurate. Many parents have the opportunity to find out the baby's sex during a routine second-trimester ultrasound scan. Although the images of the baby may be obscure to you, they are very clear to a trained eye. As long as your baby doesn't cross his or her legs, your technician or practitioner will probably be able to tell the sex. Whether he or she tells you is for you and your partner to decide. For some couples, the decision is easy; for others, it may involve some negotiating. Ray and I decided to be surprised, and we had a lot of fun wondering and imagining. But we had many friends who couldn't imagine not knowing!

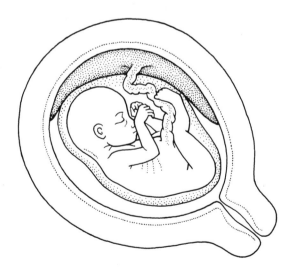

By far, the two most exciting events that happen this month are hearing your baby's heartbeat and feeling him move. Your doctor or midwife will listen with a Doppler device at each of your prenatal visits. If you try listening with the device, you will clearly hear the heartbeat, too. You will also begin to feel your baby's movements. At first, you may sense only a flutter, and you may think that you have indigestion. But in a few weeks, you will clearly feel him kicking and stretching.

Your baby is floating contentedly in his watery world. With periods of rest and sleep, he moves much of the time, extending and folding his arms and legs, twisting, and making facial expressions. He practices breathing, he swallows amniotic fluid, and now that his kidneys are fully functioning, he urinates. His urine adds to the amniotic fluid in your water bag. He gets all his nutrients and oxygen from you, through your placenta. You may notice his movements increase shortly after you've eaten, when he gets an energy boost from the rise in your blood sugar. He may react with more movement to certain foods you eat, and to sounds he hears, especially loud ones. Attending a rock concert will probably result in a very active baby! You are learning about his personality as he is living and growing inside you.

WHAT'S HAPPENING WITH YOUR BODY?

Although you probably feel more energetic than you did in the first trimester, you may be starting to experience new side effects of pregnancy. Some lucky women experience no side effects, but most women have one symptom or more.

When I hear a mom begin a sentence with "I have" or "I feel," I know she'll ask me if her symptom is normal and what she can do about it. Ninety percent of the time, my answer is yes, it is normal, here are some comfort measures, and yes, it will go away when the baby is born. Women would prefer to hear that a symptom will go away sooner, but this rarely happens. A growing baby has a colossal impact on every part of the body!

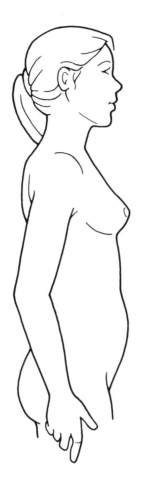

Common Discomforts of Pregnancy

The following paragraphs describe some common second- and third-trimester discomforts and some simple remedies for them. You may also experience some symptoms not listed here. If you are ever worried about new symptoms, please check with your practitioner.

HEADACHES

During pregnancy, headaches are most often caused by the tremendous increase—30 to 40 percent—in the volume of blood circulating in a woman's body and from the rising levels of estrogen produced by the placenta. The increased estrogen can cause vasodilation (widening of the blood vessels) in the head, which can cause a headache.

Here are some suggestions for treating a headache without resorting to medications:

- Eat often; low blood sugar can trigger a headache.
- Get plenty of sleep at night, and rest during the day.
- Take a warm, relaxing bath or shower.
- Lay a cool or warm washcloth over your eyes.
- Get some fresh air.

If you have had migraine headaches in the past and they are more frequent now, or if you are having very severe headaches, perhaps with visual changes, please let your doctor or midwife know immediately. Severe headaches can be a symptom of preeclampsia (page 194), a dangerous complication of pregnancy.

HEARTBURN

Two things cause heartburn during pregnancy: the relaxation of a muscular valve in the lower part of the esophagus, and the upward push of the growing uterus against the stomach. These two conditions can lead to *reflux*, the backing up of stomach acids into the esophagus. Reflux causes a burning sensation under the breastbone. Although heartburn can begin early in pregnancy, it is most common in the third trimester. Women with more than one baby tend to experience more pronounced heartburn.

Try these remedies for heartburn:

- Sit up for a time after meals. Don't eat right before going to bed.
- Eat smaller, more frequent meals.
- Avoid spicy, acidic, or greasy foods.
- Drink plenty of liquids throughout the day and especially with meals.
- Take a walk, or stretch your arms over your head.
- Use over-the-counter antacids occasionally, if you need to, to reduce stomach acid. Ask your practitioner what product he or she recommends.

BACKACHE

Occurring to some degree in nearly every pregnant woman, backache is caused by the forward pull of the spine as a woman's center of gravity changes.

You can take several measures to prevent or relieve backache:

- Be very careful when lifting anything. Always bend your knees and lift with your legs instead of your back.
- Consciously practice good posture by keeping your shoulders high, your buttocks tucked, and your abdominal muscles firm.
- Wear good, supportive shoes. If you must wear heels, do so no longer than necessary, and keep them to a height that is manageable for you. Your comfort and safety are much more important than fashion.
- Apply ice or heat when your back is sore.
- When rising from bed, always turn to your side and push yourself up with your arms.
- Ask your partner for frequent back massages, or try a professional massage. Massage is simply wonderful!
- Try pelvic tilts and pelvic rocks (page 150). These exercises can strengthen your back and abdominal muscles, which support your uterus and maintain your center of gravity.

LEG CRAMPS

These are especially common during the second and third trimesters of pregnancy. Despite the many theories about why leg cramps occur, there are no certain answers. It was formerly thought that leg cramps might be caused by a need for more calcium, but studies have not confirmed this explanation. Pressure from the baby and decreased circulation in the legs are other possibilities.

Here are some good practices to remedy leg cramps:

- Walk frequently, or do the one-minute stretch (page 124) several times a day. This exercise involves lifting and bending your knees as if you are in a marching band. Walking or marching increases the circulation in your legs.

Do the One-Minute Stretch

If you must spend most of the day sitting, taking occasional breaks for this exercise may help prevent leg cramps, swelling, and lightheadedness.

1. Stand, and lift your hands over your head, interlocking your fingers.

2. Gently stretch upward for a count of five.

3. With your hands over your head, gently lean to the right, and stretch for a count of five. Lean to the left, and stretch for another count of five.

4. March in place, bringing your knees as high as you comfortably can, for a count of ten.

5. While supporting yourself with a hand on a chair or wall, rotate your right foot clockwise for a count of five, and then counterclockwise for a count of five. Repeat with your left foot.

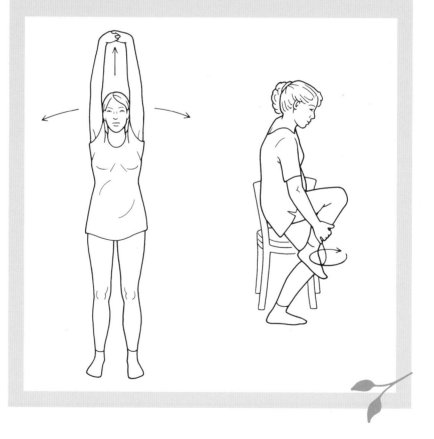

- Put your feet up as often as possible. Getting off your feet can also help decrease the swelling in your legs and feet.
- Before bed, take a warm bath or just keep your legs warm. The warmth can decrease the likelihood of leg cramps.
- Never point your toes; this position can cause an immediate cramp.
- To stop a leg cramp, flex your foot by pulling your toes toward your knee.

CONSTIPATION

The increase in progesterone during pregnancy slows the digestive system. If you are prone to constipation or are taking iron tablets (page 81), you'll want to be especially careful about your fiber and fluid intake. Many women have less trouble with constipation after they move into the third trimester.

Try these remedies for constipation:
- Drink, drink, drink. Hydration is the key.
- Eat whole-grain breads, brown rice, and plenty of fruit and vegetables. Bran and prunes are especially helpful.
- Try fiber supplements such as psyllium husk, but remember that these can increase your constipation if your fluid intake is inadequate.
- Try over-the-counter or prescription "stool softeners" if your practitioner recommends them.

HEMORRHOIDS

These are dilated veins in the rectum. In pregnancy, they are caused by increased pelvic blood flow and pressure from the baby. Hemorrhoids may bleed or hurt, especially after the baby is born. Let your practitioner know if you have any rectal pain or bleeding.

VARICOSE VEINS

Dilated blood vessels, or varicosities, sometimes occur in the legs, thighs, or vulva during pregnancy, because of increased blood flow and the compression of blood vessels by the uterus. Varicose veins can be uncomfortable, and many women are bothered by the way the veins look. The veins recede after the baby is born.

These remedies for varicose veins may be helpful:

- Try not to stand for long periods.

- Spend some time each day lying down with your feet on a pillow.

- Apply an ice pack directly on the varicosities to relieve swelling and discomfort.

- Wear support stockings.

MINOR BLEEDING OR BRUISING

Increased blood flow and hormonal changes affect the capillaries (tiny blood vessels) during pregnancy. For this reason, nosebleeds, bleeding gums, bruising, and spotting after lovemaking are normal and quite common. Still, you should let your practitioner know if you experience any bleeding in pregnancy, so you can be reassured that it is within normal limits. Some evidence suggests that a slight increase in vitamin C intake can reduce bruising.

SWELLING OF HANDS OR FEET

The dramatic increase in blood and other fluid levels during pregnancy often results in swelling, or edema, especially in the hands, feet, or both. Occasionally, the swelling exacerbates or even initiates carpel tunnel syndrome, which is characterized by numbness and pain in the wrists. Because swelling can be a sign of preeclampsia (page 194), be sure to tell your practitioner about any swelling that you experience, anywhere in your body.

These steps can help you avoid or reduce swelling:

- Keep your diet balanced. Avoid salty foods, and be sure to eat plenty of protein foods such as meat, fish, poultry, tofu, milk, yogurt, beans, and low-fat, low-salt cheese.

- Drink plenty of water. Remember your six to eight glasses every day!

- Avoid standing or sitting in one place for long periods. Take short walks frequently, or just move your legs. This is especially important when you are traveling by car or plane.

- Put your feet up several times throughout the day. It's best to elevate your feet with a pillow so that they are higher than your heart.

- Wear good, supportive shoes and support stockings if you plan to be on your feet for a long time.

LIGHTHEADEDNESS OR DIZZINESS

Because of low blood pressure, pregnant women sometimes become lightheaded or feel faint when they stand up too quickly or get out of a hot bath or shower. As discussed on pages 36 to 37, low blood sugar and anemia (low iron in the blood) can also cause dizziness or lightheadedness, so be sure to let your practitioner know if you have these symptoms, especially if you have fainted.

Try the following remedies to alleviate faintness or dizziness:

- When you feel dizzy, sit down and lower your head to your lap. This allows blood to move more easily to your brain.

- Try to move a little slower than usual, and avoid sitting or standing in one place for a long time.

- Throughout the day, occasionally exercise your calves by moving your feet in a circular motion.

- Eat frequently throughout the day.

- Keep your bath or shower at a moderate temperature, and be very careful when you get out of the tub or shower stall.

DISTURBED SLEEP

In late pregnancy, many women find it hard to get comfortable at night. They are often too hot and, of course, they must make frequent trips to the bathroom. (Interestingly, not all pregnant women need to urinate frequently. Because Alexander was positioned quite high in my body, I had no increase in my trips to the bathroom—although I felt as though my ribs were being stretched by a shoehorn!)

Two steps might help you get a good night's sleep:

- Use a lot of pillows—against your back, between your knees, in front of you. Snuggling against Dad may help, too, of course, if you are not feeling too hot.

- To reduce nighttime visits to the loo, avoid eating a heavy meal close to bedtime, and try to decrease how much you drink in the evening.

STRETCH MARKS

These are white or reddish streaks that appear most often on the breasts and abdomen. Caused by the stretching of the skin, the marks occur more frequently in light-skinned people than they do in dark-skinned people. Creams, lotions, and oils can't prevent stretch marks. The marks fade after the baby is born, although they do not disappear completely.

DRY, ITCHING SKIN

The stretching of the skin on your abdomen can cause it to become dry and itchy. Lotion can help considerably with this.

Another skin condition that sometimes occurs in pregnancy, though far less commonly (in less than 1 percent of pregnant women), is called PUPPP, or *pruritic urticarial papules and plaques of pregnancy*. It is characterized by reddish, itchy, raised patches on the skin, mostly on the abdomen, and is most common in a first pregnancy. If the rash is severe, it can be treated with medications. Although potentially quite bothersome, PUPPP is not harmful to either mother or baby, and it disappears after birth.

IMPORTANT THINGS TO KNOW

In my practice, I have found that many of my clients' unspoken questions revolved around sex. Until now, your sexual relationships affected only you and your partner. Now you may have questions about how this relationship can affect the three of you: you, your partner, and your baby.

Sex and Romance

Nearly every expectant couple experiences changes in the sexual relationship during the course of the pregnancy. If this is your first baby, you and your partner are used to being just two. Now you have added another little being to your lives. Although the baby is yet unborn, both of you are very much aware of your baby's presence. When you make love, your growing baby may be especially noticeable. Both the physical changes of pregnancy and your feelings about the baby may influence your sexual relationship. It is important to know what is typical and how to remain sexual beings even as you are growing into parenthood.

Your fuller, more radiant body is a testament to the fact that you are a sexual being. In magazines and other media these days, pregnancy is portrayed as sexy and sensual, and so it is. You may not always feel beautiful, but you *are* beautiful. Allow yourself to revel in your new beauty.

If you were fatigued and nauseated in early pregnancy, your sexual appetite may have suffered. As your pregnancy progresses and you begin feeling a little more energetic, your sexual desire will probably return, if it hasn't already. It may be stronger or weaker than it was before you were pregnant. The increased blood flow to your pelvic region and the second-trimester rise in estrogen may heighten your sexual desire, and greater vaginal lubrication may increase your sexual pleasure. Your partner may be confused by the sudden transition from the early weeks of pregnancy, when even the thought of lovemaking may have sent you running for cover, to the "I can't have enough of you" weeks of the second trimester. (When I was pregnant, my friends and I shared laughs over how our "poor, confused" husbands dealt with our changing sexual appetites. One of my friends told of times her husband pleaded for her to leave him alone!) Be assured that your baby is undisturbed by your lovemaking, although she may increase her activity in response to hormonal surges and contractions from your orgasms.

As your pregnancy continues, more changes within your body will affect your sex life. Your breasts may be tender, and after your sixth month or so, they might leak *colostrum* during sexual play (colostrum is the substance your body produces to nourish your baby in the first few days after birth, until your milk comes in). As your baby grows and your body shape changes, you may be more comfortable if you and your partner adjust your sexual positions. You may prefer to be on top during intercourse, or to lie side by side with your partner, like spoons or facing one another. Your partner may be able to feel the baby during lovemaking, and he may be unnerved by this. Reassure him, and again, change positions if this helps. If you tire easily at night, be creative with the time of day you make love. Try a romantic meeting in the afternoon, or enjoy the early morning. Help your partner to understand what is comfortable and pleasurable for you.

Because of the increased pelvic blood flow, your vagina is more engorged and there is an increase in the number of small capillaries in your cervix. These increases can cause a small amount of bleeding during lovemaking, especially with deep penetration. Vaginal bleeding of any kind warrants a call to your doctor or midwife, but a little bleeding during lovemaking is usually no cause for alarm. You may be able to avoid this bleeding simply by avoiding deep penetration.

In late pregnancy, female orgasm sometimes causes uncomfortably intense contractions that last for minutes or recur intermittently for hours. Unless you are considered at risk for preterm labor, these contractions are likely to be normal and safe. But at times, you may want to skip having an orgasm during lovemaking or just cuddle with your partner instead.

Although this is a time of change for both you and your partner, your sexuality remains an important part of the two of you and your relationship. Enjoy this time together before you become parents. Dine out occasionally, cook special meals, enjoy movies or the theater, or just take a quiet walk. If, because of vaginal bleeding or a risk of preterm labor, your doctor or midwife has advised you to limit your sexual activity, you can still cuddle and kiss without having either intercourse or an orgasm. Being together and expressing your love for each other in many ways—not just sexually—will strengthen your relationship and help you to welcome the new addition to your family.

Ask Tori, R.N.

"PELVIC REST"

Hi, Tori,

I am 18 weeks pregnant, and I have been having some vaginal bleeding and contractions. I am scheduled for an ultrasound check next week. My doctor told me that in the meantime, I should decrease my activities at home. He said something about "pelvic rest," which I thought meant no sex, but now I am not sure. I am too embarrassed to call and ask him what it means. Can you help?

—Andrea, Kansas

Andrea,

You are certainly not alone in wondering what "pelvic rest" means, or feeling uncomfortable about asking a doctor for details of what you may and may not do sexually. Being on pelvic rest means you shouldn't do anything that might cause or increase bleeding or contractions. That means you need to adhere to the following guidelines:

- *Nothing in the vagina.* This includes tampons, penis, or fingers.
- *No orgasms (for you).* They can cause contractions, so even oral sex and masturbation are out.
- *No breast stimulation.* Stimulating the breasts releases the hormone oxytocin, which can cause contractions.

Once you have your ultrasound, your doctor will learn more about what may be causing the bleeding.

ANTERIOR PLACENTA

Dear Tori,

I was told by an ultrasound technician that I have an anterior placenta. What exactly is this? Is it why the baby's heartbeat is sometimes hard to find, and why I don't feel as much movement as other women who are 19 weeks along?

Also, does my being overweight make it harder to feel the baby kicking?

—Tanya, New Jersey

Dear Tanya,

A placenta can implant in any number of places, including at the top of the uterus (the *fundus*), at the back of the uterus (*posterior*), or, in the case of *placenta previa* (page 196), in the lower portion of your uterus, covering your cervix. Having an anterior placenta means that it has implanted along the front portion of your uterus, directly under your belly button. An anterior placenta is perfectly normal, and yes, it is the reason you do not feel the baby's movements as much as other women do. Instead of kicking directly against your abdominal muscles, the baby is kicking and pushing against the placenta. This softens the impact for you, as if you were cushioned by a pillow inside. This is also why it is sometimes hard to locate your baby's heartbeat. My Alexander had an anterior placenta, and I was a bit disappointed that I did not feel him moving around much.

If you have a layer of fat on your abdomen, this further cushions the baby's movements.

STRESSED DAD

Tori,

Two months ago, we found out my wife was pregnant, and we're both very excited. I tell myself that everything is fine, but I find myself constantly worried, and I notice that I am having stomachaches and tension headaches. Does this happen to prospective fathers a lot?

—Ed, Idaho

Dear Ed,

You are not alone! A man's discovery that he is going to be a father brings up many emotions. In addition to being happy, you have new concerns. You may be worried about the health and safety of your wife and baby, the responsibilities of parenthood, household finances, changes in your lifestyle, and much more. Things that you have never worried about before may suddenly seem like looming problems. The enormous scope of fatherhood is often underestimated. Many men experience physical symptoms of anxiety as they adjust to their new role.

The good news is that your anxiety will very likely pass. In the meantime, share your feelings with your wife or a close friend.

If you find that you are continuing to worry, talk with your doctor about how you feel.

AIR TRAVEL

Dear Tori,

My husband and I are scheduled to fly for three hours to visit his family. I will be 17 weeks along, and I'm scared to death that something may happen, like turbulence on the plane, or that I'll just feel lousy the whole time. The visit will be only for a weekend, but even at home, I am uncomfortable and have trouble sleeping.

—Kimberly, Nebraska

Dear Kimberly,

If your pregnancy is normal and your practitioner hasn't told you otherwise, flying at 17 weeks should be safe. Doctors and midwives discourage air travel after 36 weeks, but this is only because of the risk that a woman could go into labor during her trip.

Your letter implies, though, that either you dislike flying or you just don't want to take this trip. Only you can decide what you'll be comfortable doing. Discuss your feelings with your husband, and if you decide to go, be sure that he will give you the support you need. Plan to take a lot of deep breaths during the flight, allow plenty of time for rest once you arrive, and relax as much as you are able. If talking with your husband doesn't relieve your anxiety, perhaps it is best to postpone the visit until after the baby is born.

SECOND-TRIMESTER MISCARRIAGE

Tori,

I have recently heard some frightening stories about miscarriages occurring in the fourth or fifth month. I thought my miscarriage worries were over after 12 weeks! I've read that sometimes the initial symptoms are very subtle, just a slight pressure and a slightly heavier discharge. Well ... how slight? I'm in my seventeenth week, and my abdomen sometimes feels heavy. I find myself wanting to hold it up. Is this just a normal symptom of pregnancy?

—Courtney, Arizona

Dear Courtney,

The thought of miscarriage is always frightening, and a little information can cause much needless worry. Very often, a brief description of a pregnancy complication in a book or on the Internet turns out to be more upsetting than useful. Although second-trimester losses do occur, they are unusual, and they are very often related to an already known problem with the pregnancy.

One possible cause of late miscarriage is preterm labor (page 170). The symptoms of preterm labor can be subtle, since the cervix can dilate, or open, and efface, or thin, with or without painful uterine contractions. But usually, these cervical changes are accompanied by frequent, rhythmic uterine contractions that feel like menstrual cramps or are more painful. Any such contractions before your 37th week of pregnancy should be reported to your practitioner.

Feeling pressure from your growing uterus is quite normal. After about 30 weeks, so are mild contractions, called Braxton-Hicks (page 162). You may also feel your uterine (round) ligaments stretching, or you may notice some fetal movement that seems different, or "tight." These normal feelings are sometimes mistaken for labor contractions.

Try not to worry about every new sensation during pregnancy. If you are concerned, talk with your doctor or midwife. He or she is a far better source of information and reassurance than your next-door neighbor or the woman in front of you in the grocery line.

Tori's Tip: Walk, Walk, Walk

Yoga, swimming, and prenatal exercise classes are all good ideas. But working out at a pool or gym or attending an exercise class is just not realistic for many women. My best suggestion for maintaining a healthy body during pregnancy is to walk. Walk as much as you are comfortable with and have time for. When the weather permits, take a daily walk outdoors. This can be a wonderful way to spend time with your partner or a good friend. If you don't have time for a long walk, refresh yourself with a couple of short strolls each day. And, when you have the choice, take the stairs instead of the elevator.

DAD'S CORNER

A lot is happening this month, and you may have quite a few questions. Common ones are "Why is my partner still nauseated?" "Is that really the baby moving?" and, finally, an important but sometimes unasked question: "Uh, is sex okay?"

Nausea. Eighty percent of women say they feel much better at 16 weeks, and very few women continue to experience nausea after 20 weeks. So, if morning sickness seems determined to claim your sweetie for eternity, hang in there! Some women say that fresh air helps enormously, and they take to eating in the backyard. For other tips on dealing with morning sickness, see page 47.

The Baby's Movements. To feel your baby move against your hand can be exhilarating. Was that a foot or an elbow? Baby gymnastics is a source of joy and amusement for both partners, especially as the pregnancy progresses and you can see your child's tiny fist or cranium slide by. Don't be surprised, however, if Mom's enthusiasm wanes as the baby's activities increase in strength and frequency.

Sex. Frequently, dads report a near to complete conversational vacuum on the topic of sexual activity during pregnancy. Hesitant questions and furrowed brows may characterize any discussions you may have. Many women, as well as their partners, are unsure about what is and is not okay.

Here is the scoop: *Unless your partner is at risk of preterm labor or has a medical condition that makes certain positions unsafe, go for it!* Sex is fun, and there is no reason that you and your mate shouldn't have the same kind of fun that you normally do. Some things will change, of course; perhaps your spouse is more easily aroused at a different time of day than she was before she became pregnant, or maybe she finds a particular position more comfortable. Be creative and honest with each other. If you need specific advice, talk with your partner's doctor or midwife.

Intimacy, sexual or not, is the key to maintaining mutual understanding and the ability and will to resolve conflicts in your relationship. And humor, both in and out of your bedroom, helps an awful lot.

Treat Her Well. Most importantly, let your partner know that she is attractive, beautiful, sexy. Use whatever descriptive words tell her how much you love her and her changing body.

Another sweet gesture is to gather a few baby pictures of both of you. (You might ask relatives for copies of ones you don't have, and so have a chance to relive childhood memories with soon-to-be grandparents or other family members.) Many new parents are astounded by how much their own baby pictures look like those of their newborns.

Enjoy the Old Wives' Tales

No doubt, you are starting to hear them. Formulas that predict the baby's sex are the most popular, perhaps because even when they have no basis in fact, they have a 50-50 chance of being correct. Here are some of my favorite old wives' tales about all aspects of pregnancy:

- If you carry high or "wide to the side," the baby is a girl.
- If you carry low or "out front," it is a boy.
- A high heart rate is a girl's, a low one a boy's. (Or is it the other way around?)
- If a needle or ring suspended on a thread over your abdomen swings clockwise, the baby is a boy; if the object swings counter-clockwise, the baby is a girl.
- If a longish piece of cotton cloth held over your abdomen moves back and forth, the baby is a boy; if the cloth hangs straight, the baby is a girl.
- Compare mom's age at conception with the year of conception. If both are even or odd, the baby is girl; if one is even and one is odd, the baby is a boy.
- If you have heartburn when you're pregnant, the baby will have a lot of hair.*
- If you crave strawberries (and then eat a lot of them during pregnancy), your baby will have a strawberry-colored birth-mark, or "stork bite."
- If you raise your hands above your head, the umbilical cord will strangle the baby.
- You can't get pregnant if you have sex standing up!

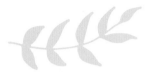

Beginning the Carefree Months
YOUR FIFTH MONTH: WEEKS 20 THROUGH 23

THE FIFTH MONTH OF PREGNANCY is the period that many women describe as the most fun. Your belly is a comfortable rising-moon shape, your baby is moving, you have heard the heartbeat, and your energy level is high. People are beginning to notice your pregnancy, and the excitement is building. You have much to look forward to in the coming months.

Your baby is growing, growing, growing. At the end of this month, she will weigh 10 to 12 ounces (283 to 340 g) and measure nearly 10 inches (25 cm) long, about the length of a large eggplant. During her waking hours, she stretches, kicks, and turns somersaults in her water bag; she still has plenty of room to move. She also sleeps a lot, as much as 20 hours a day. You may notice periods when she is extremely active and other times when she is very quiet. This is completely normal.

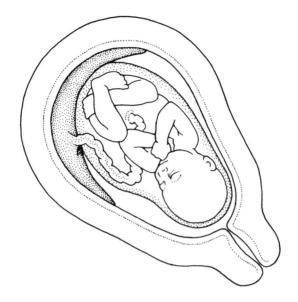

In addition to lanugo (soft, downy hair), a white creamy, protective coating called *vernix* covers her body. Her eyelashes and eyebrows are very distinct, and her facial features become clearer each day. Up until now, her head was much larger than the rest of her body, but her legs and torso are growing rapidly, lengthening her body. Her arms, legs, fingers, and toes are all fully formed, and her nails have grown to near completion. She looks much more like a baby than she did last month.

With a Doppler device (page 302), you and your practitioner can easily hear your baby's heartbeat. You could probably even hear it faintly with a stethoscope on your abdomen. Your baby's heart beats about 140 to 150 times per minute. By the time she is born, her heart rate will be anywhere between 120 and 160 beats per minute.

WHAT'S HAPPENING WITH YOUR BODY?

Putting on Pounds

Most women gain weight gradually throughout pregnancy. You probably gained 2 to 6 pounds (0.9 to 2.7 kg) during the first trimester, although some women remain at their pre-pregnancy weight or even lose pounds during this period, and this is okay. You can anticipate gaining 2 to 6 pounds (0.9 to 2.7 kg) every month during the second and third trimesters. Your total weight gain is likely to depend largely on your pre-pregnancy weight and the number of babies you are carrying (see above).

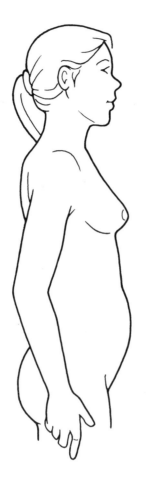

Gaining the needed weight doesn't take much effort. Before pregnancy, an average woman must consume about 2,000 calories per day to maintain her weight. During pregnancy, she needs about 2,400 calories per day. If you began your pregnancy very under- or overweight, your practitioner may ask you to count calories and pay close attention to how much you eat. But if you fall into neither of these categories, you are likely to gain the amount of weight that is right for you, just by eating nutritious foods according to your appetite. Increased feelings of hunger should drive you to take in the extra calories you need.

IMPORTANT THINGS TO KNOW

As your abdomen grows, it can be a challenge to find clothing that both looks good and feels good, whether you are at work or at play. And once you have found well-fitting casual clothes, you may want to take advantage of their comfortable fit and wear them to exercise.

Dress for Comfort with Twins

If you are pregnant with twins, you can expect to need maternity clothes much sooner than mothers of single babies do, perhaps even by the end of the first trimester. When I was expecting Alexander, I first wore a maternity shirt at around 17 weeks. I am not even sure I needed it then. By contrast, my friend Cris, who is much taller than I, was clearly showing by week 9 or 10 with her twin girls and was wearing maternity clothes by week 13. By late pregnancy, you can expect to need large- and extra-large-size maternity clothes, even if you are normally a small person.

It can get very expensive to purchase several sizes of maternity clothes that can be worn to work. Many women say that large, button-down shirts and non-maternity stretchy pants help supplement their maternity wardrobe.

You will also want to have on hand comfortable clothes for wearing around the house, especially if your practitioner suggests that you decrease your activity or requires bed rest.

Remember that comfort is always the key, even when planning your work wardrobe. You can always spruce up a simple outfit with a scarf or jewelry. Most important is that you can sit and stand comfortably in what you are wearing.

What Will You Wear?

If you haven't bought maternity clothes already, you will now probably need to get some. In recent years, designers have stepped up to create fashionable maternity clothes for work, dress, or casual wear. But many items in maternity stores and catalogs are expensive, especially considering how short a time you'll need them. Before going shopping, look through your closet and dresser. You may have baggy shirts, loose dresses, and stretch pants that you can wear through most or all of your pregnancy. Talk to any friends or relatives who have recently had babies; they might have some nice things that you could borrow. Check whether your community has a store that sells gently used maternity and baby clothing. When you start shopping, keep comfort and practicality in mind, and consider buying some items that you'll want to wear after the baby is born.

When selecting clothes, too, consider which season you'll be wearing them in. Will you need them in warm weather or during the cold winter months? I was so excited when I went shopping for maternity clothes that I bought a beautiful, sleeveless, silk "dressy" dress. Alexander was born in December! I recently gave the dress to a friend, having never worn it.

What follows is some more specific advice, compiled from comments I've heard from many moms over the years as well as from my own experience. Have fun shopping for the new, temporary you!

BRAS

Not only do your breasts enlarge during pregnancy, but your rib cage expands as well. Some women wear their old bras throughout their pregnancies, but most women need to buy a couple of new ones in a larger size. To be sure that your new bras will continue to fit until your baby's birth, I suggest using a maternity or department store with expertise in fitting pregnant women.

Choose bras that are both supportive and comfortable. Avoid underwires, even if you usually prefer them. They may feel too constrictive during pregnancy, and they shouldn't be worn when breastfeeding, since they can cause the blockage of milk ducts. You may find that you perspire more now and that synthetic fabrics aren't comfortable, so favor cotton.

You might buy a nursing bra if you plan to breastfeed, but to ensure a proper fit, you are probably better off waiting until after your baby is born and your milk has come in; your breasts are likely to be even larger then. For example, I went from a size 36 to a size 38 during pregnancy, but my cup size went up, from A to B, only after Alexander was born (in truth, I was probably really an AA before I got pregnant!).

UNDERPANTS

Some women keep wearing their bikini panties through pregnancy, but as your abdominal girth increases, you will probably want to buy maternity underpants. There are two types: The first fits below your abdomen, and the second comes up over your abdomen. You might try one pair of each and then decide which is more comfortable. Again, cotton is best.

If you are used to wearing thong underwear, you may find that panties, or at least a wider thong, are more comfortable now.

SWIMSUIT

If you are going to spend time at a pool or beach over the next few months, you may want to get a maternity swimsuit. Maternity stores have a wide selection, or a friend may have a little-used one to lend you. If you normally wear a bikini, you can keep on wearing it. I always love seeing a pregnant belly in a bikini.

PANTS AND OVERALLS

Comfortable pants for pregnancy have a drawstring or elastic waist. Pants sold as maternity wear usually have an elastic panel that stretches over the abdomen; even jeans are available this way. There are also maternity overalls, though many women find that they can wear a regular pair of overalls through most of their pregnancies.

You will probably want three or four pairs of casual pants and at least one pair of dress pants. If you must dress up for work, you may need more maternity slacks. Remember, though, that you will use these clothes for only a short time. It is less expensive to vary your outfits with tops and scarves than to purchase numerous suits or dresses.

EXERCISE PANTS AND SHORTS

Stretch knit workout pants are easy to find and very comfortable to wear with big sweaters, oversized shirts, or tunics. A few pairs of stretch pants may be sufficient for your entire pregnancy. Many women wear them instead of maternity pants.

Bicycle and workout shorts are available with stretch maternity panels. If you are not active in sports or will be delivering in the winter or early spring, you probably won't need workout shorts at all.

SHIRTS AND SWEATERS

Generally, men's shirts and oversized, or "plus" size, tunics, smocks, and sweaters work very well. You can wear these throughout your pregnancy and long after the baby is born, and you don't need to spend a lot of money for them. If you would like dressier blouses, visit a maternity store for the best selection.

DRESSES

Unless you have to dress up for work, one or two dresses will probably be plenty. Maternity shops have the best selection of formal dresses, but each piece can be expensive. Oversized, loose-fitting dresses not designed specifically for pregnancy often work very well.

TIGHTS AND PANTYHOSE

You will probably need to buy some new stockings if you wear dresses, especially in cold weather. You can move into queen-size tights or pantyhose or buy stockings designed for pregnancy at a maternity shop. Support hose may make you more comfortable if you have any swelling in your legs.

SHOES

A little-known fact is that many women's feet become larger during pregnancy and often stay that way forever after (my shoe size was 7½ before pregnancy; it is now a solid 8). Even if your feet don't spread, any swelling can make your shoes uncomfortable. If you buy new shoes, you'll probably need a half-size larger than usual. Make sure that they are supportive and comfortable. Even for the most fashion-minded women, wearing heels higher than 1¼ inches (3 cm) during pregnancy is just not fun! For warm weather, a slide-in (backless) sandal may be very practical.

OUTDOOR COAT

Your winter coat may allow enough room to accommodate your growing belly. If not, you may get by with heavy sweaters or one of your partner's jackets. If you have to buy a new jacket or coat, make sure it's one you'll want to wear after the baby is born.

How, and How Much, to Exercise

Why do I keep bringing up exercise? Exercise helps all of us feel better, physically, mentally, and emotionally. It burns calories to prevent excess weight gain, keeps our muscles and joints strong, and lowers our risk of heart disease and other serious illnesses. For pregnant women, exercise also has been shown to decrease the incidence of gestational diabetes, a form of diabetes that develops during pregnancy (page 193). Additionally, when you exercise, you gradually develop the stamina required for labor and birth and, in the early postpartum period, for the physical demands that new motherhood brings.

The American College of Obstetricians and Gynecologists says,
"Unless there are medical reasons to avoid it,
pregnant women can and should try to exercise moderately
for at least 30 minutes on most, if not all, days."

Watch That Stretch

During pregnancy, the hormone relaxin makes your pelvic joints—and all your other joints—looser and more flexible in preparation for birth. Some pregnant women say their joints feel wobbly. Because your joints are more flexible, it is possible to overextend them, causing injury. Be careful when you are stretching!

Physical exercise has also been shown to decrease the incidence of postpartum depression. During exercise, the body produces less of the stress hormone cortisol and more of the calming neurotransmitter serotonin. Women who exercise regularly are more likely than others to report feeling accomplished, confident, and positive about life.

I don't want you to feel that if you don't go to a gym, you aren't exercising. To me, exercising means keeping your body moving. If you are healthy and your pregnancy is progressing normally, it is not only safe but also beneficial for you to be active. What kind of exercise you do doesn't matter, as long as you do something physical for 20 to 30 minutes at least three times a week. Even a daily 10-minute walk is beneficial.

Moderation is key, however. Aerobic activity tends to become more difficult as pregnancy progresses. Stop exercising if you become breathless, lightheaded, overheated, or just tired; never exercise to the point of exhaustion. Keep your heart rate at 80 percent of your maximum or no higher than 140 beats per minute. If you were lifting weights before pregnancy, it's fine to continue, but to avoid back strain, you will need to modify the way you use them as your center of gravity changes. If you do sit-ups, bend your knees to help avoid the separation of the abdominal muscles, an uncomfortable though not dangerous condition. Always include a warm-up and a cool-down period when you exercise. Drink plenty of water. And be sure to stretch, stretch, stretch!

Tori's Tip: Do Some Simple Exercises

These exercises are helpful anytime, but especially during pregnancy. You can do them as frequently as you like.

Pelvic Toning (Kegels)

Kegels (named after the gynecologist who developed them) are exercises in which you squeeze and then relax the muscles of the perineum, the area between your vagina and anus. The perineum will stretch when your baby's head passes through your vagina at birth. Doing Kegels can help tone these muscles in preparation for your baby's birth and help you to recognize the difference between holding your perineum tight and relaxing it. Kegels are even more important after your baby is born, when they can help the perineal muscles recover. The exercises also help prevent urinary incontinence. As we age, the muscles that support the bladder, uterus, and vagina can weaken. Making Kegels a lifelong habit can keep these muscles toned throughout the rest of your life.

The easiest way to learn how to do Kegels is on the toilet. Begin to pee, and then stop your urine midflow. You are tightening your perineal muscles. Begin to pee again. You are relaxing the muscles.

You can do Kegels in any position—sitting, standing, or lying down. Do about ten each day. Choosing a particular time to do them may make it easier to remember them.

Pelvic Tilt or Pelvic Rock

The pelvic tilt is an excellent exercise to relieve back discomfort and strengthen your lower back. Move into a hands-and-knees position with your back flat. Smoothly roll your hips forward toward the floor while keeping your shoulders and upper back still. Straighten again. Remember to inhale and exhale slowly and keep your movements slow and steady.

You can also do this exercise while standing against a wall or lying on your back on the floor. While standing, press your lower back into the wall, and then release. While on your back, with your knees bent and a pillow under your head, press the small of your back into the floor, and then release.

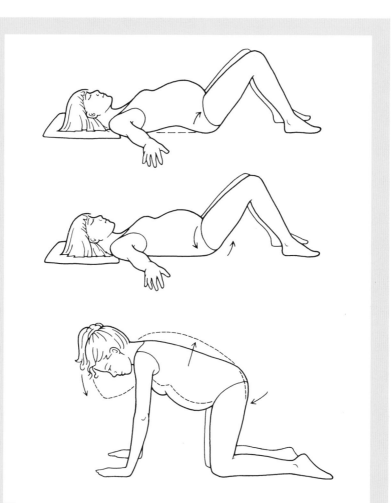

Arched Cat

The arched-cat position can help relieve upper body tension and the pressure you may feel in your back from your enlarging belly. Move into a hands-and-knees position as you did for the pelvic tilt, with your back flat and your head and neck straight. Then arch your back as a cat does, pulling your hips forward and lowering your head. Close your eyes, and keep your inhalations and exhalations full and relaxed. Hold for a count of three, and then return to your original position. Do this several times a day.

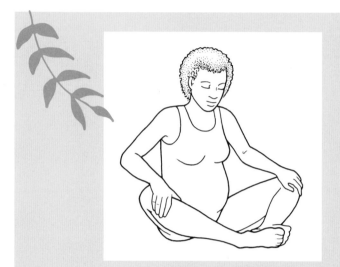

Tailor Sit and Stretch

This exercise opens your pelvis and stretches your inner thighs, shoulders, arms, and upper back. Sit cross-legged on the floor, and slowly raise your hands above your head. Stretch one arm and then the other up to the sky. Repeat 10 to 20 on each side.

Many pregnant women find it comfortable to sit cross-legged even when they are not exercising.

Neck and Shoulder Rolls

Slowly roll your head two to three times, first clockwise, then counterclockwise. Repeat several times. Next, raise your shoulders up, and roll them backward for a count of five, then forward for a count of five. Repeat this several times.

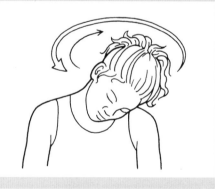

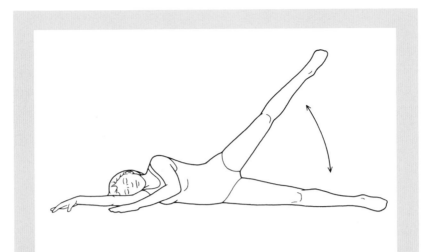

Leg Lifts

This exercise strengthens your inner thigh muscles. Lie on the floor on your side, aligning your head, shoulders, hips, and bottom leg. You can either bend your top leg and rest it on the floor in front of you or keep it straight. Lay your head on the floor, or prop it up with your hand. Place your other hand in front of you for support. Slowly raise your top leg to a comfortable height, keeping the leg straight and your toes flexed. Hold this position for a moment, and then lower your leg. Do this ten times on each side, and then repeat.

If you have had an exercise regimen in place since before pregnancy, you can probably continue it, although you should check it out with your practitioner. Your changing body may limit your ability to continue some athletic activities. You'll want to avoid sports in which you could be hit in the abdomen, such as kickboxing or soccer. Sports that require a great deal of bouncing, such as jogging or aerobic dancing, can be replaced with activities such as low-impact aerobics, vigorous walking, or swimming. Sports that are more adventurous, such as downhill skiing and horseback riding, are no more dangerous during pregnancy than at other times, but they could pose unnecessary risks of injury to both you and your baby. Use common sense, and follow your body's cues.

A terrific way to get exercise and meet other moms-to-be is to join a prenatal exercise or yoga class. These classes include a variety of physical exercises and stretches adapted for the pregnant woman. Ask other pregnant women or new moms for recommendations, or check with your local hospital, community college, YMCA, or YWCA.

Here are some sensible and safe exercises to do throughout your pregnancy:

Walking. This easy-to-do exercise increases your circulation, maintains your endurance, combats fatigue, and strengthens your muscles in preparation for labor.

Swimming. The benefits of swimming are the same as for walking. In addition, floating in the water makes you feel weightless; you can move freely despite your expanding belly.

Stretching or yoga. These exercises increase your flexibility, promote relaxation, and can relieve back pain and improve posture. Prenatal yoga classes exclude certain poses that may not be safe during pregnancy. Yoga is a wonderful way to slow down and center yourself while getting a good workout.

Pilates. This exercise method involves a series of controlled movements that strengthen the whole body, increase flexibility, and improve concentration, breathing, and body alignment. Pilates originally involved specialized machines; today, however, the exercises are often done with just a mat. I suggest working with a Pilates instructor who is familiar with pregnancy, because some exercises may be unsuitable for this time.

Aerobics and dance. Low-impact aerobics is fine as long as you are comfortable with it. Dance of all kinds is wonderful exercise during pregnancy, but avoid a lot of jumping and bouncing.

Bicycle riding. Cycling is a terrific aerobic, non-weight-bearing activity that you can do outdoors or on a stationary bicycle.

Relaxation routines. Audiotape relaxation exercises can teach you where you hold your tension and how to release it. This skill can be helpful when you are in labor.

DAD'S CORNER

While your partner's belly is beginning to resemble a mountain, a mountain of other things are happening. People are beginning to treat the two of you as parents, you're making plans for life with your baby, and you may have questions about the health of the baby and your partner. New concerns can pile up quickly beside your everyday concerns about work and the household. Let's see how to reduce that mound to molehill size.

Be involved. If you haven't yet been along on a prenatal checkup, go when you can. If you have concerns or questions, write them down, even if they seem trivial, and take along the list. Your mate's body is doing things mysterious to both of you, and the more you understand intellectually, the easier it is to connect with her emotionally. Most moms are delighted when their partners show interest in the pregnancy.

Learn. Read this book! Spend a little time finding baby information on the Internet, and watch the Baby Channel once in a while. Your mate will love it!

Help your partner and your baby stay healthy. Help her to eat healthy foods and to exercise. Take walks together, go for a bicycle ride, play tennis, or go dancing.

Help plan for the baby. Talk to your partner about what both of you want for the baby. Decide where he will sleep, and help arrange the room. Shop together for the baby's things. It may seem early, but now is the time to buy any new furniture, because it could take several weeks to arrive.

Treat Her Well. Make an intimate ritual of measuring your partner's belly. You might buy a cloth tape measure and write the date at each weekly measurement with a permanent marker. In a few years, your child will love to see how fast she grew.

Buy your partner a book that has nothing to do with babies or pregnancy—a good mystery, maybe, or a collection of short stories. Too much reading about pregnancy can be overwhelming and entirely unhelpful. Both of you may need a break from all this information.

Whether you pick up a novel or *The Joy of Pregnancy*, it is nice to sit in bed and read aloud to each other. Ray and I did that with a lot of books, and it was always a very special time together.

Ask Tori, R.N.

BABY'S MOVEMENTS

Hello, Tori,

I am 25 weeks pregnant, and sometimes I feel my baby move very little or not at all. Other times, he seems to move constantly. Is this normal? How do I know that he is okay?

—Samantha, South Dakota

Samantha,

Babies have activity cycles just as we do. They can be more active or less so at different times of the day. Within an hour, they will have, on average, one 20-minute sleep cycle. They move more during the hour or so after Mom has eaten a meal, in response to the rise in her blood sugar. You may notice a few more punches, rolls, or kicks during that time.

Many women say that they feel their babies move the most at night. This could be because the baby starts moving when you stop or because you simply notice the baby's movements more when you slow down.

Kick Counts

If your doctor or midwife has asked you to count your baby's kicks, record how long it takes to feel ten movements. Begin counting soon after a meal, when the baby is likely to be active. Counting ten movements should take no more than two hours, and it will probably take less time.

If ever you question whether your baby is moving, please check with your doctor or midwife.

CAN I LIFT THINGS DURING PREGNANCY?

Tori,

My husband and I are transforming our spare room into a nursery. I will need to do a lot of lifting, although it won't necessarily be heavy. Is it safe to do this? Will there come a time when it is no longer okay?

—Amanda, Oregon

Dear Amanda,

There is no time when lifting is absolutely safe or unsafe. If you aren't under any medical limitations, you can follow these guidelines.

During the first trimester, you can do whatever you did before your pregnancy. For example, if you were comfortably able to lift 30 pounds (13.6 kg) before, then you could still do so, unless you are feeling too fatigued. Good body mechanics and back-saving techniques are always important: Bend at the knees rather than the waist to lift a heavy object.

During the second trimester, you will probably feel more energetic, so this may be the best time for projects such as rearranging the furniture and decorating. You can lift things carefully, keeping in mind that your center of gravity has changed and that you will be less balanced in certain positions. I recommend against lifting any amount of weight that causes you to strain.

During your third trimester, it is best to leave the lifting to others. You need to reserve your energy and strength, and at this stage, it is much more difficult to maintain balance when lifting. If you must lift something heavy, have another person help you, and never lift more than you comfortably can.

Many couples move or take on remodeling projects shortly before a baby is born. If you are going to be moving into a new home or renovating the current one, it's best to get resettled a couple of months before the baby arrives. If you must take on a physically demanding project in late pregnancy, obtain as much help as you can get. You might invite over a group of friends, supply the pizza and sodas or beer, and have a party while getting the heavy work done. This can make for some happy memories after the baby is born.

PREGNANCY AND THE FLU SHOT
Hi, Tori,

I am 22 weeks pregnant and healthy, but I am a bit concerned that I may get sick during the winter months. I usually get a flu shot. Should I get it this year or skip it?

—Jennifer, Nevada

Jennifer,

Yes, you should get the flu shot this year. Pregnancy can decrease your immunity and so put you at increased risk of getting the flu. Pregnant women are also at greater-than-average risk of developing serious complications of the flu, such as pneumonia. If you were to get the flu when your baby was a newborn, your baby might get it, too.

The vaccine contains three influenza viruses that have been identified as likely to cause widespread infection in a given year. Your body takes about two weeks after you receive the vaccine to develop antibodies to the influenza viruses. Knowing that the flu season is at its height from December through March, the Centers for Disease Control and Prevention recommend that pregnant women be vaccinated in September or October.

Because the flu vaccine is made from killed (inactivated) influenza viruses, it is considered safe during any stage of pregnancy. There has been concern regarding the very small amount of thimerosal, a mercury compound, in the flu vaccine, but we have no convincing evidence that this preservative poses a risk to either mom or baby. The primary side effect of the vaccine, for pregnant women as for others, is minor swelling and redness at the injection site.

You may have heard of a nasal-spray version of the vaccine that is sometimes given instead of a shot. The spray is made from weakened (attenuated) live influenza viruses, and so I don't recommend it for pregnant women.

To keep yourself as healthy as possible through the winter and throughout your pregnancy, maintain a nutritious diet, drink plenty of fluids, take your prenatal vitamins, and get adequate rest.

LOW-LYING PLACENTA
Dear Tori,

My obstetrician has told me that I have a low-lying placenta. What exactly does that mean? Will I need to have a cesarean section?

—Heather, Tennessee

Heather,

In the early stages of pregnancy, as the embryo settles into the uterus, the placenta usually forms in the upper portion of the uterus. This area is called the fundus. With a low-lying placenta, however, the placenta forms in a lower portion of the uterus. This is a problem only if the placenta covers all or part of the cervix. If the entire cervix is covered, the condition is called *placenta previa*. It is not safe to deliver the baby vaginally when the mother has placenta previa, since the passing of the placenta first could cause serious bleeding in both mom and baby. In this case, a cesarean is needed.

Generally, however, a low-lying placenta moves up and away from the cervix as the uterus expands. Although the placenta is attached to the uterine wall, the expanding uterine muscle shifts the placenta upward.

Because a low-lying placenta can cause bleeding, your doctor may have already placed you on "pelvic rest" (page 131). You will have an ultrasound scan later in your pregnancy to determine where your placenta is positioned. If it is out of the way of the cervix, you can resume your normal activities, including sex, and you can expect to deliver your baby safely vaginally.

ROUND-LIGAMENT PAIN

Hi, Tori!

I am 23 weeks pregnant. A couple of weeks ago, I lifted my four-year-old and had a very painful, stretching feeling in the middle of my abdomen. I called the doctor, who said that it was probably the ligaments that hold up my uterus stretching. A few days later, the pain happened again, several times, when I would stretch or move in an unusual way. Now it happens when I walk the dog or reach for something, or even when I am sitting still. It feels like a spasm, and it actually makes me jump! Do you think I should call the doctor again?

—Tracy, Ohio

Dear Tracy,

It sounds to me as if you are experiencing *round-ligament* pain. On both sides of your uterus are ligaments, called *round ligaments*, that help to support it. As your uterus grows, these ligaments stretch. The stretching may cause a sharp twinge or pain when you move suddenly, turn, cough, or sneeze. The pains often occur over a period when a baby is having a growth spurt. Round-ligament pain is perfectly normal and nothing to worry about. It is another one of those uncomfortable conditions of pregnancy that will go away as soon as the baby is born.

WHERE DOES THE BABY'S URINE GO?

Dear Tori,

I'm having a little girl, and I'm very excited! My question is a little embarrassing: When my baby urinates or has a bowel movement, where does this waste go? Is it floating around in the sac with her?

—Wendy, Texas

Dear Wendy,

The truth about embarrassing questions is that they often are the ones *everyone* has. Anything that passes through the baby's body ends up being part of the amniotic fluid.

Your baby's urine is made up of products different from ours. The more urine your baby produces, the more amniotic fluid you have.

Since your baby is not digesting any food, she is not yet having any bowel movements. Shortly before birth, however, your baby may pass a bowel movement in your womb. This first stool, called *meconium*, is very sticky and dark green. Meconium is ordinarily first passed in the initial few hours after birth. A baby's passing of meconium before birth can mean that she is postmature (past 41 weeks' gestation) or has been under some kind of stress. If you notice a greenish or dark yellowish vaginal discharge, please let your practitioner know. This could mean that your water bag has broken and that the baby has passed meconium. Your doctor or midwife will want you to come into the hospital or birth center, so that you can be checked.

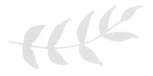

Planning for Birth
YOUR SIXTH MONTH: WEEKS 24 THROUGH 27

YOU ARE NOW MORE THAN HALFWAY through your pregnancy. But you already knew that. As you move further along, you of course move closer to giving birth to your baby. This month, we'll talk about some concerns you may be having and what plans you may want to set into motion.

WHAT'S HAPPENING WITH YOUR BABY?

This is a very exciting month in your baby's growth. Scientists believe that during this time, a baby becomes aware of his environment. This means that he becomes responsive to sounds, such as music and your voice. Your baby may become more active when he hears loud music or sudden sounds and quieter when he hears your voice or soft music. Soon he will see a little, too. His eyelids will part this month, and his eyes will open for short periods. There is some evidence that once a baby opens his eyes, he can faintly see light through his mother's abdomen.

Your baby is just over 1 foot (30 cm) long now, and he weighs 1½ to 2¼ pounds (680 to 1,020 g). His skin is translucent, as it has very little fat underneath it. This month, his own distinct tiny handprints and foot-prints develop. His growth from this point on will be quite dramatic.

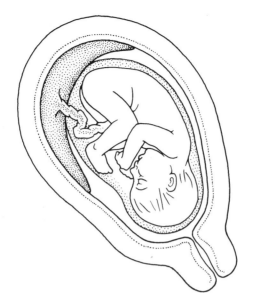

He still has plenty of floating room in the amniotic fluid. This fluid allows him to grow and move freely and serves as a cushion in case your belly gets bumped. When I was seven months pregnant with Alexander, I tripped and fell directly on my belly as I was hurrying across the street. Neither of us was hurt. I felt as though I had fallen on top of a rubber ball!

Your baby will continue to produce amniotic fluid up until the moment he is born. Years ago, people incorrectly believed that if a mother's water bag broke early in the labor, there would be no more amniotic fluid and the baby would have a "dry birth." But when the fluid sac breaks, during or before labor, the fluid continues to be produced.

If your baby were to be born during this month and could be cared for in a neonatal intensive care unit, he would have a chance of surviving. Medical science, however, has not yet been able to reproduce the amazing work of your placenta. The umbilical cord, made up of three vessels—two arteries and one vein—is the baby's lifeline. Oxygen and nutrients from your blood pass through the placenta and on to the baby through the umbilical vein. Once the baby uses the nutrients, the umbilical arteries carry carbon dioxide and waste products away from the baby, and your body eliminates them. Although the placenta filters out certain substances and viruses, most things pass easily through. Essentially, everything that enters your body also enters your baby's.

WHAT'S HAPPENING WITH YOUR BODY?

The first time you notice your belly tightening, you may mistake this nonlabor uterine contraction for the baby's movement. Such contractions are called Braxton-Hicks, after John Braxton-Hicks, the doctor who studied them. They are thought to prepare the uterine muscle for labor by toning it and promoting blood flow. Compared with the contractions you will have in labor, Braxton-Hicks are mild, but they may feel quite strong when you put your hands on your belly. Though irregular and painless, these contractions can be uncomfortable. They may be triggered by the baby's movement, someone's touching your belly, an orgasm, a change of position, a need to urinate or have a bowel movement, or being dehydrated. A Braxton-Hicks contraction stops when you change your position or activity; for example, if you start feeling a contraction while you are lying down, it will end when you stand up. If the contractions bother you, drink a tall glass of water or take a warm bath or shower. Some women experience Braxton-Hicks contractions regularly, and others never notice them at all. Either situation is perfectly normal.

Should You Call the Doctor?

If you ever experience uterine or back pain that is regular, repetitive, or painful, let your practitioner know immediately.

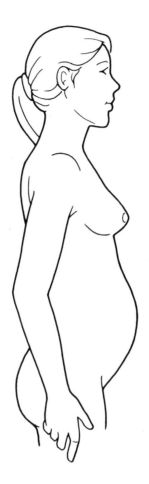

Although Braxton-Hicks contractions can begin in this second trimester, they are more common in the third. Once they have begun,
they will continue throughout the rest of your pregnancy.

These contractions have no effect on the initiation of labor or dilation of the cervix, but when they occur close to delivery, they can help
soften and efface (thin) the cervix. Strong and frequent Braxton-Hicks
contractions are sometimes referred to as "false labor" (page 272).

IMPORTANT THINGS TO KNOW

At 6 months, planning for birth is not just a hypothetical activity. Now is the time to enroll in a childbirth class. And although preterm birth is quite rare, you might read over the later section pertaining to this topic. Knowledge of what to do in the unlikely event that you begin your labor early can help you feel relaxed and confident during this enjoyable time in your pregnancy.

Classes for Parents-to-Be and New Parents

Before the mid-twentieth century, the most help a woman could hope for in preparing for birth was some wise advice from her mother, sister, or friend. Fathers were not involved in birth at all. For many women, giving birth for the first time was frightening. Childbirth education has radically improved the experience of childbirth for most women.

Depending on where you live, you may be able to choose among many types of classes for parents-to-be and new parents. Some places offer classes as narrowly focused as "Pregnancy Meditation" and "Preparing for Twins or Triplets." Here are some typical offerings:

Pregnancy planning. Usually taught by a gynecologist or nurse-practitioner, these classes cover fertility, conception, and caring for your health before and during pregnancy.

Early pregnancy. Most often taken during the first trimester, these classes cover information about changes in a woman's body, fetal development, and nutrition. Because so many women have a small library of pregnancy books at home, many communities are eliminating early-pregnancy classes.

What Was Your Birth Like?

It may be fun to hear your parents tell about your birth. What was your mother's labor like? What was the experience like for your dad? What do they remember most?

Take a Tour!

If you are taking your prenatal class at the hospital where you will be giving birth, the class may include a tour. Some hospitals offer separate tours. In either case, a tour is an important part of your preparation for birth. It is comforting and helpful to see where you will be having your baby, and to ask questions of the staff.

Prenatal exercise. These classes are led by a physical therapist or a personal trainer with advanced training in obstetrics, the musculoskeletal system, and women's health. The classes generally include low-impact aerobics, stretching and strengthening exercises, and relaxation. For safety, most of these classes require a doctor's referral.

Prenatal yoga. These classes are designed to increase comfort and flexibility in a pregnant woman's rapidly changing body; to alleviate common discomforts of pregnancy such as back pain, sciatica, swelling, anxiety, and fatigue; and to help the woman connect with her developing baby. Many women find prenatal yoga classes to be both relaxing and energizing.

Labor and childbirth preparation. These are most often designed as a series. There is instruction in relaxation and breathing to reduce the discomfort of labor, massage, positions for labor and birth, the partner's role, hospital procedures, medicated and non-medicated labor, anesthesia, and cesarean birth. You and your partner will want to take a course taught by a certified childbirth instructor, a registered obstetrical nurse, or a midwife.

Breastfeeding. A certified lactation consultant discusses the benefits and basic techniques of breastfeeding; how to prevent, recognize, and manage difficulties; and how partners can help.

Refresher for childbirth or breast-feeding. For those who already have one or more children, these classes provide a review and an update of labor and birth, breathing and relaxation methods, and the partner's role during birth and breastfeeding.

Newborn parenting. These classes can be great fun, as they often involve hands-on practice (on dolls) with diapering, wrapping, dressing, and bathing. Newborn appearance and behavior, infant development, and practical tips for new parents are frequently included.

Infant safety and CPR (cardiopulmonary resuscitation). I recommend that parents take one of these classes when their babies are 3 to 6 months old, although the demonstrations and practice are on infant mannequins rather than real babies. The classes address how to recognize and treat emergencies such as choking and respiratory difficulties, how to perform basic first aid, how to "childproof" a house, and how to avoid common childhood accidents.

Infant massage. These are wonderful classes to take with your baby. They teach gentle massage strokes that promote digestion, elimination, and relaxation in the early weeks after the baby's birth.

New moms' support groups. These informal groups, a lifeline for many new mothers, often sprout from a childbirth preparation class. Although dads are usually welcome, the groups tend to be made up primarily of women whose babies are close to the same age. Sleep, husbands, work, sex, all things baby, and life in general are discussed.

I started a new moms' group when Alexander was born, and the other women have become some of my dearest friends. We call ourselves the Sanity Sisters. We do things together with our children as well as without them. We try to have dinner out at least once a month, and we occasionally even include spouses! For nearly five years, the kids spent every Wednesday together, and they now think of each other as cousins. Today, there are twelve children between the six of us. I have heard similar stories about such friendships from mothers everywhere.

Support groups for parents of multiples. I strongly recommend that moms of twins and other multiples get dialed into their local twins or multiples mothers' support group while they are still pregnant. These groups can be an enormous help. Depending on where you live, you may find one or more groups. Because urban areas tend to have a lot of twins, if you live in or near a city you may have several groups to choose from. In your local community, first check with your own hospital or childbirth education center. Time and again, I hear women say that they wish they had become involved in a multiples group before their babies were born. They feel that the chance to talk with a mother who had been through the experience would have saved them from having to figure it out alone.

Here is a very telling quote from a mother of twins: "I figured that I was an efficient, high-energy career woman, that I didn't need any special support, and that I would figure out what was best for our family. But once the twins came, it changed everything. I realized that I couldn't just 'figure it out.' My parents-of-multiples group helped me find a much-needed night nurse to help care for my children from 10 P.M. to 6 A.M., twice a week, so that I could get some sleep. This was an expensive indulgence for us, but worth every penny. I was so exhausted that I could barely function, and my night nurse was my savior! Later, I went to a couple of the multiples-club support groups, and ended up meeting two moms who remain close friends to this day."

CHILDBIRTH-PREPARATION CLASSES

Of all the classes just described, the most important for first-time parents is a class on preparing for labor and birth. Although it can be helpful to read books and watch a video or two on birth, books and videos don't provide enough information to help you fully understand labor or learn effective coping skills. Taking a class will help you learn as much as you can about your new adventure (never forget that this is a wonderful adventure!).

There are many benefits to taking a childbirth-preparation class. The most important is that you will gain a realistic expectation of what will happen during labor and birth. What's more, you will learn various coping mechanisms and gain confidence in yourself.

Some childbirth-preparation classes teach one childbirth "method" or another. To help you understand the differences between these schools of thought, I'll give you a brief history. In the late 1940s and 1950s, women were often heavily medicated in labor, and they were alone. Their husbands were not welcome to participate, and there were no doulas (page no 249). Women spent at least seven days in the hospital after giving birth. These practices led to a strong, much-needed movement to bring childbirth back into the family.

At this time, a physician named Grantley Dick-Read identified something he called the fear-tension-pain cycle. Dick-Read believed that a lack of knowledge makes laboring women afraid. Fear creates tension, tension increases pain, and pain makes us more afraid. Through this cycle, fear, tension, and pain escalate. Dick-Read developed a way to use information and relaxation to break the fear-tension-pain cycle. All the childbirth "methods" subsequently developed were intended to manage this cycle.

During this same period, two other physicians, Ferdinand Lamaze and Robert Bradley, developed their own philosophies and methods of preparing women for labor. Although there are a few additional methods, such as the Alexander technique, which reteaches the body how to move, think, and release tension, and hypnobirthing, which uses relaxation and repeated positive statements, most childbirth classes emphasize either the Lamaze or the Bradley approach. Both of these popular methods advocate particular breathing and relaxation techniques for labor. With each approach, a woman is "coached" or supported by her partner or another caring person.

The basic Lamaze philosophy is this: By understanding the labor process and by learning specific relaxation and breathing techniques, you can decrease the pain associated with labor contractions. By learning how to focus outside your body (for example, on a picture), you will be better able to cope. Today's typical series of Lamaze classes, completed over several weeks or a weekend, lasts 10 to 12 hours.

The Bradley method, originally referred to as "husband-coached delivery," teaches natural childbirth, without medical interventions. Typically 12 weeks long, the training focuses on nutrition, exercise, and deep abdominal breathing for labor. According to Bradley, tuning in to your body, rather than focusing outside it, is the best way to cope with pain. Although Bradley instructors address the use of medications, the disadvantages of medications are emphasized over the advantages. In my experience, the Bradley breathing and coping techniques are excellent for women who want to labor without medications, but the critical view of hospitals often presented in Bradley classes may create unnecessary tension for couples choosing hospital birth.

One current method of using focused breathing and relaxation as a way of managing the process of labor is called "hypnobirthing." It is not appreciably different from previous forms of natural labor coping techniques. Hypnobirthing focuses on visualization, deep breathing, and the use of music, as well as quiet verbal prompts of positive feelings by those supporting the laboring woman. Much like I recall from Ina May Gaskin's wonderful book *Spiritual Midwifery*, contractions are referred to as "surges" or "waves."

Today, childbirth-preparation classes often incorporate the best aspects of various childbirth methods, although many emphasize basic focused breathing techniques. Whether you will be having your baby in a hospital, a birth center, or at home, I recommend that you attend a class that teaches the following things:

- *Physiological aspects of labor and birth*—what happens and when.
- *Coping skills*—relaxation, breathing patterns, massage, focus, and other ways to minimize pain in labor.
- *Labor support measures*—working with your body through positions, movement, and other natural ways to foster the process of labor.
- *The partner's role*—how your mate can support you and work with the rest of your team.
- *Accurate, unbiased information* on the use of medications, monitoring the mother's and the baby's well-being, and the circumstances in which medical procedures are needed. Even if you are planning a home birth, it is important to understand why transfer to a hospital might be needed and what might happen when you are there.
- *Cesarean birth* (page 304)—not only why this might be necessary but what to expect should you need one. I tell my classes that a mother "gives birth" whether she does so vaginally or by cesarean section.

With most of us so busy these days, many childbirth-education programs offer a variety of scheduling options. You can select a weekly evening class, a weekend class, or even an abbreviated one-day course. I know of some weekend classes that are held at a resort, so that couples can combine childbirth education with a weekend getaway. If you are on bed rest, have an especially busy schedule, or just want personal attention, you can also ask about private classes.

Because some classes are very popular, you should sign up soon to be sure of getting a place. But you don't need to start the course right away; you will best retain what you learn if you take your class shortly before the birth. Unless the baby comes prematurely, the birth will occur between 37 and 42 weeks' gestation. Seventy-five percent of women, in fact, deliver between weeks 39 and 41. So I recommend planning to complete your course by your 37th or 38th week.

Many organizations and individuals offer childbirth-education classes. Your obstetrician or midwife may recommend a particular teacher or program but may not know about every class available in your community. Before choosing a class, think about what is important to you: Do you want to learn a particular philosophy or technique, such as the Bradley method or hypnobirthing? Do you want to take a class at the hospital or birth center where you'll deliver, so that you can learn more about what to expect there? After considering your preferences, ask your friends for recommendations, check with a local community college or the hospital or birth center where you'll have the baby, or look in the yellow pages. You can also try looking on the Web for classes in your local area.

Preterm Labor

Labor that begins earlier than 36 weeks is considered preterm. It is defined by uterine contractions that are strong enough to cause the cervix to efface and dilate prior to term gestation. Occurring at 20 to 36 weeks' gestation, preterm labor precedes almost half of preterm births and is the leading cause of neonatal mortality in the United States.

Although some practitioners treat for preterm labor whenever a woman is having rhythmic, persistent contractions, these are sometimes actually *prelabor*, or Braxton-Hicks, contractions (page 162).

Tori's Tip:
Choose the Childbirth Class
That's Right for You

Here are some questions you might ask before choosing a childbirth-preparation class:

- Who sponsors the classes—the hospital or birth center where you'll deliver, a separate organization, or an individual?
- What are the instructor's credentials? Is the person affiliated with any organization? At PillowTalk, all our instructors are registered nurses who work with moms and babies in hospitals. Midwives, certified childbirth educators, and doulas can also be high-quality instructors.
- Does the class advocate a particular philosophy? If so, what is it? Does the approach seem practical and objective?
- What topics are covered in the class?
- How does this class differ from others offered in the area?
- How many couples are in each class? I recommend taking a medium-size class, with 10 to 12 couples.
- Can you bring more than one support person?
- Can you come alone?
- Where is the class held?
- How many meetings are in each series of classes, and how long does each meeting last? Are there different options for class times, such as evenings, weekends, or all day?
- What is the cost for the class? Will your health insurance cover any of the cost?
- Do you need to bring anything with you?

If you are expecting twins or more, check to see if there are any classes in your area especially designed for women and families expecting more than one baby. These classes often discuss the specific concerns around a multiple's labor, birth, and new-baby period.

Preterm labor can begin without any noticeable contractions. The following are common signs that labor is beginning:

- Low back pain, or pressure and heaviness in the pelvis
- Menstrual-like cramps that are regular and may be painful
- Reddish or brownish mucous discharge from the vagina
- Watery discharge, either a sudden gush or continuous leaking over a few hours

If you experience any of these symptoms, let your practitioner know right away.

Preterm labor can be diagnosed with certainty if a woman's cervix has begun to soften, thin, or dilate. These cervical changes can be identified and measured through ultrasound. If you are undergoing cervical changes with or without contractions, your practitioner will try to stop labor until your baby reaches a safer gestational age, 36 weeks or more.

Preterm labor is more common in multiple gestations. The incidence with twins is approximately 50 percent and, with higher-order multiples, 70 percent or more. The average length of gestation for twins is between 35 and 37 weeks.

Women at risk for delivering early are now frequently identified by a test for *fetal fibronectin* (fFN), a protein that is produced during pregnancy but that doesn't normally appear in the vagina after 22 weeks' gestation. Between weeks 22 and 34, a sample of cervical secretions is taken in the same way that a Pap smear is taken. If fFN is present, the membranes may be breaking apart, and a preterm delivery could result.

Can Preterm Labor Be Stopped?

Usually, yes. Being diagnosed with preterm labor means your body has begun the labor process early. It does not necessarily mean that your baby will be born early!

CAUSES OF PRETERM LABOR

Since we don't know exactly what causes labor to begin at all, it is hard to say why labor sometimes begins early. We know that the statistical risk is increased by multiple gestation (twins, triplets, or more), an abnormality in the baby, drug or alcohol abuse or chronic illness in the mother, prior miscarriage or previous premature birth, or a problem with the uterus, cervix, or placenta. But sometimes a woman with a perfectly normal pregnancy and no risk factors experiences preterm labor.

TREATMENT FOR PRETERM LABOR

Several levels of medical interventions can be used to try to stop a labor that has begun too early. Usually, the first step is to get the woman off her feet for a time, through bed rest (page 176). Relieving the vertical pressure on the cervix and minimizing her activity may be enough to quiet things down. The challenge with bed rest is that the mom generally feels perfectly healthy and is disinclined to rest all day, day after day.

Some women experience more than one miscarriage or preterm birth. Recent studies have shown that taking the hormone progesterone, either vaginally or by injection, can decrease or prevent uterine contractions, which may prolong a pregnancy. There is also a classification of medicines called *tocolytics* used to treat preterm labor.

Magnesium Sulfate (MgSO$_4$): This intravenous medication is the most common tocolytic used today. It relaxes the muscle tone of the uterus, which can prevent or decrease contractions. It also has been shown to provide neuro-protection if a baby is born prematurely.

Nifedipine: Although it is used primarily as a cardiac medication, it has also been shown to be the most effective oral tocolytic with the fewest side effects.

Indomethacin: This is an excellent medication for women who experience preterm labor before 30 weeks. Because it can decrease the amount of amniotic fluid around the baby, it is generally not used for more than three days.

Another drug given to women in premature labor is **betamethasone**, a corticosteroid that stimulates the maturation of the baby's lungs. Premature infants whose mothers have been given corticosteroids are more likely to survive and have a lower incidence of respiratory distress

Tori's Tip:
Make the Best of Bed Rest

If your practitioner prescribes bed rest, here are some ideas for managing the experience:

Set up your space. Put a cooler at your bedside. In the morning before your partner goes to work, have him put your lunch, snacks, and plenty of water and other cold drinks in it. If possible, have your laptop or tablet in front of your perch, and a table at your side. On it, you'll keep the following items:

- Any medicine you must take
- *The Joy of Pregnancy* book
- Two nonpregnancy books, different enough to suit your changing moods
- Your cell phone or home phone and easy access to phone numbers
- A player for music and audio books
- A variety of magazines of whatever your interests are

Start a project. Design your baby's birth announcement; even address and stamp the envelopes. Learn a new hobby, like knitting or crocheting. Start a journal; this may be hard to believe, but later on, it will be fun to look back on this time. Study a foreign language

and bleeding in the cranium, two of the most severe consequences of premature birth. Betamethasone is given as two injections over 12 to 24 hours. The beneficial effects take approximately 48 hours to develop.

A woman in premature labor may remain at home, monitored by her practitioner or a home monitoring service, or she may be admitted to the hospital. As long as her cervix has not dilated significantly and her amniotic sac remains unbroken, her pregnancy can probably be maintained to full term.

through books, recordings, and the Internet. You can do amazing things while lying on your side!

Binge watch and listen. If you can afford a service such as Netflix, Pandora, or Audible, now is a great time to catch up on all those shows you've heard about, listen to new music, or take in an audible book. It can really help pass the time.

Socialize. Put the word out to family and friends that you would like visitors—just to hang out, to watch a movie, or to play cards. Write letters to family and friends. Send e-mail or instant messages to keep in touch with folks.

Amuse yourself. Get good at solitaire. Subscribe to a Hollywood rubbish magazine. Work the newspaper's daily crossword or sudoku puzzle. Paint your toenails and fingernails, ask a friend to do this, or schedule an in-home professional pedicure.

Pamper yourself. Schedule an in-home weekly massage, if you can afford it, or enlist Dad. If friends ask how they can help, have them do a load of laundry or bring you a home-cooked meal. Feel free to nap!

Mark off each day of your pregnancy on your calendar.

Always remember that you are doing the important job of helping to keep your baby safe inside.

Ask Tori, R.N.

BED REST

Tori,

I have been diagnosed with pregnancy-induced hypertension, and I have been placed on "strict bed rest." What exactly does that mean?

—Christina, Colorado

Dear Christina,

Pregnancy-*induced hypertension* is an older term that is sometimes used interchangeably with *preeclampsia* (page 194). If you have high blood pressure and not the other symptoms of preeclampsia (swelling and protein in the urine), your doctor may refer to your condition as chronic *hypertension*. Any of these terms means that your blood pressure is too high.

One in five pregnant women spends a week or more of her pregnancy on bed rest, as treatment for any of several things—preterm labor, vaginal bleeding, placenta previa, preeclampsia, chronic high blood pressure, sciatic pain. A milder treatment for some of the same conditions is "decreased activity"—staying home most of the time, avoiding exercise, and putting your feet up for a while several times a day. Bed rest is usually prescribed with a qualifying term— *partial, moderate,* or *strict.* The following guidelines typically accompany the prescription:

Partial bed rest. For part of the day, you can be out of bed and moving about the house, but for the remainder of the day, you must be horizontal, lying on a couch or bed. You may be told to be off your feet by a certain time of day.

Moderate bed rest. You must lie on your side, either in bed or on a couch, for most of the day. You can take a quick shower, either daily or every other day, and eat your meals sitting up (on the bed or couch, not at the table). You must not make dinner, put a load of laundry into the washer, or do any other chores.

Strict bed rest. This is by far the most difficult. You must remain in bed (or on the couch, if your doctor approves) at least 23 hours a day. You are allowed a shower only every other day, and you must remain on your side throughout all your meals. Your food, drink, and anything else you may need must be brought to you. You can get up very briefly to use the bathroom or a bedside commode, but not for any other reason. If you are at home on strict bed rest, remember that your next stop is the hospital! Knowing this may help you follow the rules at home.

Your doctor or midwife may have his or her own particular rules regarding bed rest. Follow your practitioner's specifications; your health and your baby's health may depend on it.

NIFEDIPINE FOR PRETERM LABOR

Hi, Tori,

I'm having a minor panic attack! I have just been prescribed full bed rest and Nifedipine because of preterm labor. My doctor assured me that this is an appropriate, safe medication, but someone on an e-mail list told me that Nifedipine is not approved by the U.S. Food and Drug Administration for use by pregnant women. Is this true? Now I don't know what to think, and I'm terrified that my baby might be harmed by this medication. Please help!

—Danisha, Washington

Danisha,

Nifedipine is a medication used to treat high blood pressure and is called a Calcium Channel Blocker (CCB). Your uterus is a large, smooth muscle. Calcium is able to enter the muscle cells in the uterus, causing it to tighten. By blocking calcium from entering the cells, the uterine muscle stays relaxed.

Nifedipine is safe to take during pregnancy and has no side effects for your baby. However, because it is used primarily to treat high blood pressure, it can cause your blood pressure to lower. This may cause symptoms such as a strong headache or feeling dizzy, faint, and nauseated. Your doctor will monitor your dose very closely to prevent a decrease in your blood pressure.

DEPRESSION AND ANXIETY

Tori,

My wife is 24 weeks pregnant with twin girls. She is 41 years old, and we have a 3-year-old boy through natural conception. The twins were conceived through in-vitro fertilization.

My question is this: My wife is very depressed and anxious, and her obstetrician has prescribed Ativan, in what he describes as a very low dose. Is this common, and is it safe? My wife's family has said that she should just "snap out of it." How can I deal with them, and how can I assure her that she will be okay? Prior to this pregnancy, she never had these kinds of problems.

—Joseph, Oregon

Dear Joseph,

Depression or anxiety before, during, or after pregnancy is a real medical condition that can happen to any woman, for a wide variety of reasons. Your wife might be feeling extremely overwhelmed at having twins when she already has a young child. Also, the powerful pregnancy hormones her body is producing may be causing major mood changes. People who have not experienced severe depression often have difficulty understanding it. The actor Tom Cruise brought attention to this problem in 2005, when he publicly criticized the actress Brooke Shields for using medication to treat postpartum depression. Like many people, Cruise mistakenly believed that natural remedies and positive thinking could always cure depression. Fortunately, outcry in the media over his gaffe brought much-needed attention to this serious disease.

Ativan, or lorazepam, is an antianxiety drug often used briefly in pregnancy. Especially if the dose is low, the benefits probably outweigh the risks. I strongly suggest, however, that your wife ask her obstetrician for a referral to a mental-health professional, who will have more expertise in current treatments for depression and anxiety. Talking with another woman who has experienced depression during pregnancy or after birth might be very helpful for your wife as well.

As for your wife's family, you can tell them that a person can't just "snap out" of depression and that the condition can be life threatening. Remind them that your wife is under a doctor's care, and assure them that she is being helped.

SCIATICA

Hi, Tori,

Could you tell me a little about sciatica in pregnancy ? What causes it? What makes it worse? What helps eliminate it? What can you do to keep it from flaring up? Once you get it, does it last the entire pregnancy? And why do you only get it on one side or the other? Mine began at 22 weeks. At first, it felt like just a burning sensation in the buttocks, but if I do much walking, I also get shooting pains down my leg.

—Lindsay, Florida

Dear Lindsay,

Sciatic pain—or sciatica, as it is sometimes called—is probably one of the most painful conditions associated with pregnancy. Your sciatic nerve is the largest nerve in your body. It passes from your pelvis on either side and down the back of your thigh, where it divides into smaller nerves. You can pinch and injure the nerve in many ways; during pregnancy, however, compression of the nerve from the baby's position is the most likely cause of sciatic pain. You are probably feeling the pain on the side where the compression is.

Although you can't prevent sciatic pain, you may notice that certain positions and activities will either aggravate it or make it better. Sciatica can be completely debilitating when it flares up. Warm or cold packs, physical therapy exercises, pillows under your hip, and lying with your hips elevated may all help to relieve the discomfort, though none of these is a sure bet.

Sciatica usually does not last throughout the entire pregnancy; it often disappears completely when the baby changes position. If this doesn't happen, your sciatic pain should resolve completely when the baby is born.

THE IMPORTANCE OF CHILDBIRTH CLASSES

Hi, Tori,

I've been receiving conflicting opinions concerning childbirth classes, specifically Lamaze. I am 6½ months pregnant with my first baby and would like to know your views on the subject. Is a program like Lamaze helpful if I'm planning to use an epidural? I am from Sweden, and in my country, this doesn't seem to be such a big issue. I don't want to take the classes just because it's expected.

—Filippa, Alaska

Dear Filippa,

All labor involves some pain. Even though you wish to have an epidural, it is very important to learn about alternative ways of dealing with labor pain, and books simply cannot teach you the coping skills the way a class can. Whether your childbirth class involves Lamaze breathing and relaxation techniques or other approaches to childbirth, the class should incorporate discussions of natural methods of coping with pain as well as medication options.

As with all types of education, childbirth classes are taught by some great teachers and some not-so-great teachers, but in general these classes are extremely helpful as preparation for labor and birth. Your course should help you understand what will happen with your body in labor and how to work with this natural process. Your teacher should tell you what you need to know so that you won't be afraid of what your body is going through and so that you can make informed choices in labor. The classes provide this information in an open, accepting atmosphere in which you feel your questions are welcome. A good instructor will teach you to be flexible, because labor is always somewhat unpredictable, and will help you to feel supported, confident, and capable. By taking the classes, you will be better prepared to have a positive birth experience, whether you end up giving birth vaginally with an epidural, having a non-medicated birth at home, or having a planned or unplanned cesarean. Finally, by emphasizing that there is no right or better way to give birth, your instructor will dispel any anxiety or guilt you may feel about your choices.

PETS

Dear Tori,

As a cat owner, I have heard about toxoplasmosis, but I'm wondering what other risks animals may pose for pregnant women or infants. We have a dog and two cats.

—Shannon, California

Dear Shannon,

Pets pose few dangers during pregnancy or childhood. Of course, they must be kept healthy and clean. Dogs and cats should be appropriately vaccinated. All the animals must be friendly and safe for children to be around, and even a friendly dog shouldn't be left alone with a baby or toddler. Animals that do not tolerate children well should not be part of a human family. Most cats pay little attention to a baby. Your cats need to know, though, that the baby's bed is not a place for them to be. Once your baby is crawling and walking, make sure that the litter box is tucked away somewhere where he can't get to it. As your child grows, teach him to wash his hands thoroughly after handling any pet.

Lastly, enjoy your animals. They are a part of your family, and by growing up with them, your child will learn to love all of nature's creatures.

DAD'S CORNER

The sharing of your experiences with good friends, close relatives, or support groups can be invaluable during pregnancy, as at other times. But parents-to-be, and in particular pregnant women, are magnets for unsolicited and sometimes annoying advice. Suddenly, even strangers may feel compelled to instruct you and your partner in how you ought to live your lives.

Pregnancy is such a miraculous time that people want to be a part of it. Some may feel worried for you and believe they can help you. And still others may be unsure of how they measure up to you as a parent-to-be or partner, and so they criticize out of insecurity. Many couples hear comments like these: "Wow! Is that just one baby in there?" "Geez— you are so small; is everything okay? You really should eat more meat!" Your partner may hear dire warnings not to exercise, travel, or "think too much."

Even if these gems come from your parents or co-workers, you'll want to be firm about your boundaries. But being confrontational every time won't do you any good. You have every right to protect yourself, your partner, and your child from stressful intrusions, but the softer the interaction the better. So cool your urge to shout at the busybody in the supermarket, "No, I didn't know that polka dots could induce labor, and I'm sure no sane person does, either!" Often just a smile and a word of acknowledgment leave people satisfied to have said their piece. My advice is to be considerate, say thanks, and go on with your life. If niceness fails and someone persists in taking up your partner's time, always give your partner the chance to handle the situation herself.

Treat Her Well. Give her a trip to her best-loved quiet place—the beach, the river, a park—complete with a meal or treat. The hectic pace of our lives takes a huge toll on us and on our relationships. Your tiny, wonderful baby will bring new stress to your relationship with your partner and great demands on both her time and yours. So relax and enjoy this special time before you two are three (or four, or more).

Tori's Index

Since I am a statistics junkie, I want to share some interesting facts about today's babies and mothers in the United States.

- The average age of today's first-time mom is 27 years.
- More babies are born on Tuesday than on any other day of the week.
- The highest percentages of births occur during the morning and midday hours.
- Births on Saturday and Sunday were more likely to occur in the late evening and early morning hours than births Monday through Friday.
- Over 80 percent of women seek prenatal care during the first trimester.
- The average weight gain in pregnancy is 30 pounds (13.6 kg).
- Ninety-eight percent of babies are born in hospitals, and 9 percent of these births are attended by nurse-midwives.
- Thirty-five percent of babies are born to single moms.
- Two million of the nearly four million babies born each year belong to families with incomes below the poverty line.
- Thirty-two percent of babies are born by cesarean section.
- The rate of twin births has increased 76 percent since 1980.
- Twenty to forty percent of labors are induced, having more than doubled in the last decade.
- Twelve to twenty percent of women smoke during pregnancy.
- The months with the highest rates of birth are August, September, and October. January and February have the lowest rates.
- Forty-nine percent of newborns are girls; 51 percent are boys.

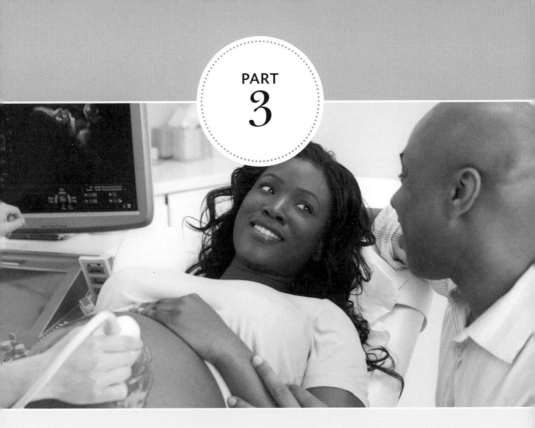

THE THIRD TRIMESTER

Planning for Life with Baby
YOUR SEVENTH MONTH: WEEKS 28 THROUGH 31

THE SEVENTH WAS MY FAVORITE MONTH OF PREGNANCY. Just like many other women at this time, I felt good; you probably feel good, too.

Around this time, your breasts may be leaking a small amount of the "premilk" substance called colostrum. This is normal and happens to many women. Later in the third trimester, you may experience discomforts related to increased size—that is, the size of both your baby and your own belly. But now, at the beginning of the trimester, you still have room to grow and you probably aren't yet very uncomfortable with that little being who is pushing against your bladder or your ribs. The seventh month is also when you may be fixing up the baby's room or enjoying a baby shower. Electricity is in the air!

WHAT'S HAPPENING WITH YOUR BABY?

Your baby has doubled her weight since last month; now she weighs just about 3 pounds (1.4 kg). She will now gain weight dramatically until she is born, and by the end of this month, she will be almost 18 inches (46 cm) long. She may have a full head of hair already, and she is beginning to develop a bit of fat under her skin. She is interacting a lot with her environment, opening and closing her eyes, perhaps sucking her thumb, hiccupping, stretching, and moving. She can hear and perceive light and shapes.

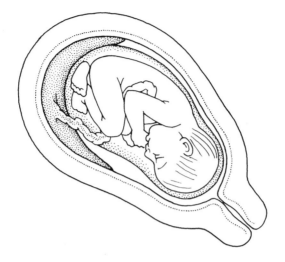

If she were born this month and could be cared for in a neonatal intensive-care nursery, she would have a fighting chance of growing to be a healthy child. But she grows faster in your uterus than she would in the outside world. For each day she remains inside you, she would need to stay two days fewer in the hospital if she were born prematurely.

WHAT'S HAPPENING WITH YOUR BODY?

Let's talk about veins. Around the seventh month is when these beauties tend to "pop up."

Varicose Veins

More common in women than in men, varicose veins often run in families. Statistics on how often varicose veins occur in pregnancy are unavailable, but about 50 percent of women will have some varicose veins by the time they are fifty. Smaller varicose veins, or spider veins, occur when tiny capillaries weaken, most often on the legs and ankles, and show up as fine bluish, reddish, or purplish lines under the skin. The increased blood supply in pregnancy can exacerbate spider veins. Larger varicose veins are swollen and bulging. Either large or small varicose veins may surface for the first time or worsen during late pregnancy, when the uterus exerts greater pressure on the veins in the legs. Varicose veins may not cause any discomfort, or they may be quite painful. Compression stockings (support hose) can provide some relief. After the baby is born, varicose veins usually become less pronounced, but they do not always go away entirely. The most common ones to remain are the spider veins.

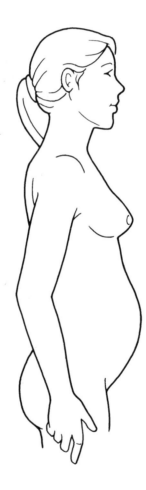

Varicose veins in the larger veins of the thighs and labia are caused by pressure of the baby's head. Although lying down can sometimes mitigate this pressure, there is no way to prevent these varicose veins. Most women find them only mildly uncomfortable and are more bothered by how the veins look. Fortunately, these enlarged veins go away after the baby is born.

Vascular Spiders

Spider nevi, or vascular spiders, usually arise only during pregnancy. These are not the same as the tiny varicose veins that are sometimes called spider veins. Vascular spiders look like tiny, red, raised lines that branch out from the center, like a spider. They appear most often on the upper body, face, and neck and are caused by the increase in estrogen. Unlike varicose veins, spider nevi cause no pain or discomfort, and they generally fade, sometimes completely, after delivery.

IMPORTANT THINGS TO KNOW

Now is the time for a little work and a little fun. By work, I mean reading over the material on special challenges. Again, these conditions are uncommon but manageable; a basic understanding of them is useful for all moms-to-be. And this month's fun—if you like shopping—comes from gathering the baby items you will need. With the myriad choices facing you, this activity is something you and your partner can do together.

Special Challenges

Although every woman hopes to have a normal, easy pregnancy, sometimes there are difficulties. The following sections discuss the most common special challenges of pregnancy.

MULTIPLES: TWINS, TRIPLETS, AND MORE

As you may have noticed, the rate of twin births has increased dramatically since around the mid-1990s. Treatments for infertility, including fertility drugs and in-vitro fertilization, are the primary reasons for the increase, although fertility centers throughout the country are now taking advantage of new technology that allows for a higher pregnancy success rate with fewer embryos. Of course, many multiple births occur naturally, especially to older mothers, women of African descent, and women with twins in the family. The potential to bear fraternal twins can be hereditary when a woman inherits the gene for hyperovulation, which causes a woman's ovaries to release more than one egg at a time.

For moms, being pregnant with twins brings higher risks of gestational diabetes (page 193) and preeclampsia (page 194). For babies, the primary risks are preterm labor and premature birth. Most twins are born two to four weeks before the mother's due date. Triplets and bigger sets of multiples tend to be born even earlier. Premature babies can have significant health problems and may need to be cared for in a neonatal intensive-care unit (NICU). The closer to their due date the babies are born, the lower their risk of long-term problems. To help prevent premature birth, a woman pregnant with twins may spend some of her pregnancy on bed rest.

If you are pregnant with twins, your practitioner will discuss with you the option of either delivering your babies vaginally or having a cesarean section. The particulars of your own pregnancy, including the positions of the babies, will determine which birthing method is the safest. Even if you plan a vaginal twin birth, a problem arising during labor may make your doctor decide to do a cesarean instead. If you have triplets or more, the crowding in your uterus and the various positions of the babies and their umbilical cords will make a cesarean section the only safe way to give birth.

Help. If you can afford it, I strongly recommend that you line up help before the babies arrive.

Even if you have a very supportive spouse and family, help still matters. The amount of outside help you line up will depend on what you can afford, but nearly all the mothers of twins with whom I spoke recommended a four-hour block once a day or at least three times a week. Having a block of time can allow you to take a power nap or do grocery shopping and other errands. Nighttime help is also extremely

Pregnant with Twins: One Mom's Story

My friend Cris shares what she learned from having twin daughters:

"The first clue that I might be carrying more than one baby came when I got an hCG [human chorionic gonadotropin, page 34] test to confirm my pregnancy. I had just missed my period, but my hCG level was already a whopping 394. My doctor suspected twins and mentioned that I could be carrying even higher-order multiples. Twins were okay with me, but the thought of more than two babies made my knees shake. We soon confirmed with ultrasound that I was carrying two fetuses. I remember asking the doctor to double- and triple-check!

"In my first trimester, I was bone-tired and positively ravenous. Some pregnant women crave protein—beef, chicken, and other meat. Not me—all I wanted was Fruity Pebbles, orange juice, and bagels. At work, I'd close my door and take a ten-minute catnap on the floor. I had never been so tired in my life.

"I had an MAFP [alpha-fetoprotein, page 99] test, and both Tori and my doctor explained that false positives are more common with twin pregnancies. My result was positive, so I had amniocentesis a couple of weeks later. Fortunately, it showed that both babies were fine.

"In the second trimester, I felt great and had tons of energy, but I was worried about the possibility of preterm labor. It's easy to dwell on all the scary things that can happen with multiples. I read one book with images of baby footprints at 22 weeks, 24 weeks, 26 weeks, and so on. I still remember how tiny those footprints were at 22 weeks. There was also a chart that showed the babies' head circumferences at various points in gestation. These pictures were unnerving; it was amazing to see how much of a difference every week makes. My advice is to be very careful what books you read. It's good to be informed, but it's not good to be paranoid.

"Because it was hard to get comfortable at night with my enormous belly, I started sleeping with a body pillow. Before I got the pillow, I was comfortable only on my back. The body pillow helped me get comfortable on my side.

"I experienced an incredible amount of movement in the last trimester. With twins, of course, there are four arms and four legs. I felt as if I were carrying an octopus when both babies moved at the same time. The movement was also very frequent, because while one baby was sleeping, the other might be wide-awake.

"It became very hard to breathe in late pregnancy, as the babies were really pushing on my diaphragm. It was especially hard to breathe when I was sitting.

"Really, the only perk of that big belly was that it made a very convenient table to rest my plate on when eating! It is too hard to lean forward to reach the real table when you're that big. It also became hard to eat much in one sitting—there just isn't much room for food when you're sharing your body with two growing babies.

"With all the weight up front, my balance changed. Once, when I was folding laundry, I leaned forward to grab a towel from the basket and did a face plant, landing with my huge belly in the basket. I needed help from my husband to get out of the basket!

"When my first daughter was born and I gave her a kiss, my nurse handed her to my husband. Oh, yes! But I wasn't done yet, I realized. A couple of minutes later, my second daughter was born. As soon as my doctor made sure that all was okay with me, I was able to hold them both. I will never forget that feeling.

"If you are pregnant with twins, my best advice is to keep your sense of humor. You will need it throughout the pregnancy, and especially once the babies come."

valuable. Some families divide their nighttime help into three- or four-hour "shifts." For example, dad takes 10 P.M. to 1 A.M., mom takes 1 A.M. to 4 A.M., and then another person (perhaps grandma) takes 4 A.M. to 7 A.M. By the time you feed each baby, change the diapers, and get the little ones back to sleep, you're pretty much awake for your whole shift. Mom may be able to pump milk for another person to use when this helper is "on call."

More on help. Do accept all offers of help: dinners, lunches, baby-sitting, you name it. This is the time to collect on all those random acts of kindness you yourself have done. If you have no family nearby, con-tact your local twins club for the names and numbers of experienced caregivers for you and your babies.

GESTATIONAL DIABETES

To meet her growing baby's need for sugar, or glucose, a pregnant wom-an's body undergoes metabolic changes that reduce the effects of insu-lin, a hormone that normally keeps blood glucose at a constant level. Sometimes these changes result in excessively high levels of glucose in the mother's blood. Gestational diabetes mellitus (GDM) is a condition of pregnancy in which a woman's body does not efficiently control in-sulin, the hormone that maintains normal levels of blood sugar. High blood sugar in the mother passes through the placenta to the baby and can cause serious complications such as pre-term labor, a large baby, and maternal high blood pressure.

There's been a significant increase in the number of women devel-oping GDM in the last ten years. The potential pregnancy complica-tions and the increased risk of a mother developing type 2 diabetes in the future have altered the way gestational diabetes is managed. Recent research has shown the importance of tightly controlling the range of a mother's blood sugar levels by diet alone or by diet and additional insulin.

GDM is first suspected if glucose appears in your urine during one of your prenatal visits or is elevated in your blood during a one-hour glucose tolerance test. In this test, done between 24 and 28 weeks' ges-tation, you drink a very sweet preparation and then have a blood sample taken an hour later. If your blood sugar tests high, you will take a three-hour test. Again, you will be given a sweet drink, and your blood sugar will be tested every hour for three hours. If the results are abnormal, you are diagnosed as having gestational diabetes. You might also have some symptoms—increased thirst, frequent and abundant urination, and fatigue. Unfortunately, these may be difficult to differentiate from general pregnancy symptoms.

Gestational diabetes can frequently be well controlled with a very healthy diet and close observation by a medical practitioner. Your practitioner will likely refer you to a special program that can teach you how to manage your diabetes. You will learn what types of foods to eat, how to test your blood sugar, and, if necessary, how to take insulin.

Tori's Tip: Don't Worry!

I cannot overemphasize that the vast majority of pregnancies occur without serious difficulties. If you do have problems during your pregnancy, the high quality of obstetrical care today will ensure good, safe treatment for you and your baby.

PREECLAMPSIA

This rather mysterious and potentially dangerous condition of pregnancy was once known as toxemia, and researchers still think that for some reason, the placenta becomes toxic to the mother with preeclampsia. The placenta may also not function as well, which can reduce the baby's growth in the uterus.

The causes of preeclampsia are unknown. But you are at a higher-than-average risk of developing the disease if any of the following conditions apply:

- This is your first pregnancy.
- You are carrying two or more babies.

- Your mother or sister had preeclampsia or eclampsia (see below).
- You are over 40 or under 20 years old.
- You are obese.
- You already have high blood pressure, kidney disease, or diabetes.
- You smoke.

Preeclampsia affects several of the body's organs and functions. The primary symptoms are generally threefold: sudden weight gain or excessive swelling of the feet, hands, or face (all from fluid retention); an increase in blood pressure (sometimes dramatic, sometimes subtle); and protein in the urine. These can result in secondary symptoms— visual changes, headaches, severe abdominal pain, and decreased kidney and liver function. There may also be changes in the body's ability to clot blood. If left untreated, preeclampsia can progress into more severe eclampsia, which is characterized by seizures in the mother and is life threatening to both mother and baby.

Usually, preeclampsia is discovered in its earliest stages. If the mother is nearing her due date and the baby's lungs are sufficiently mature, the doctor may want to induce labor. If it is too early to safely deliver the baby, the mother is treated with bed rest or medications or both, and sometimes hospitalization. Although the reason is unclear, most women diagnosed with the condition are well treated with bed rest alone. Until the baby is born, the mother's blood pressure and blood values are checked frequently, and the baby's well-being is followed by ultrasound (page 96) and fetal monitoring (page 302). If the condition of the mother or the baby deteriorates, labor is induced or a cesarean is performed, even if the baby is premature. Preeclampsia generally resolves completely within 24 to 48 hours after birth.

If you are diagnosed with preeclampsia or considered at risk for it, be sure to follow your practitioner's recommendations. With regular prenatal care, preeclampsia is usually caught early and treated successfully, and a healthy mother and baby result.

On page 308, you can read about my personal experience with preeclampsia.

PLACENTA PREVIA

This unusual condition occurs when the placenta lies in the lower portion of the uterus, covering or partly covering the cervix. The danger is that when the cervix begins to dilate, the placenta could separate from the uterine wall. The separation could lead to hemorrhage (extremely heavy bleeding) and a reduction in the baby's blood and oxygen supply.

Having a "low-lying" placenta early in your pregnancy doesn't necessarily mean you'll have placenta previa. Normally, as the uterus grows, the attachment site of the placenta moves up, away from the cervix.

Tori's Tip:
Ask for the Shower Gifts You Want

Baby showers are great fun and a terrific way to start collecting baby items. Before your friends and relatives go shopping, though, it's a good idea for you and your partner to decide what things you might like and need. Listen to advice from others, but then go into stores and see for yourself what is available. Try out equipment such as strollers; what may be useful for one family may be impractical for another. Register at a baby store or two. This will save on the number of items you'll choose to return later and ensure that you'll receive some gifts you really need.

In addition to the items listed on 201 to 223, here are some things you might ask for:

- Diaper service, if you are using cloth diapers (one month or more)
- Breast-pump rental
- Lullaby and baby music collections
- Books on infant care
- Books on child growth and development (my favorites are *Touchpoints: Birth to Three*, by T. Berry Brazelton; *Caring for Your Baby and Young Child: Birth to Age Five*, by the American Academy

Placenta previa is usually discovered when a woman has bright red, painless bleeding that may increase with activity or contractions. This can happen anytime during pregnancy, but most often occurs early in the third trimester. *If you experience vaginal bleeding in your pregnancy, it is very important to notify your practitioner immediately.* Many times, a small amount of vaginal bleeding is not a sign of a problem, and most women who experience bleeding will ultimately deliver healthy babies. Nevertheless, you should err on the side of safety and contact your practitioner if you notice any bleeding. An ultrasound will confirm the position of the placenta.

of Pediatrics; *The Baby Book*, by William Sears and Martha Sears; *Healthy Sleep Habits, Happy Child*, by Marc Weissbluth, M.D.; *Your Baby and Child: From Birth to Age Five*, by Penelope Leach; and *The Girlfriends' Guide to Surviving the First Year of Motherhood*, by Vicki Iovine)

- Classic picture books or story books
- Handmade keepsakes, such as a pillow or towel embroidered with the baby's name, a needlepoint pillow, or a cross-stitched plaque
- A handmade quilt or afghan
- Gift certificates for dinner out, food delivery, babysitting, house cleaning, or massage (for Mom)
- Homemade dinners for the first couple of weeks after the baby is born
- Footprint and handprint kits
- Hand-painted wooden alphabet letters that spell out the baby's name
- A photo album or scrapbook and related supplies

To prevent possible further bleeding, a woman with placenta previa needs to remain on bed rest (page 173) for the remainder of her pregnancy. She may be hospitalized or carefully monitored at home until the baby is mature enough to be born safely. Because it is not safe for the placenta to emerge before the baby, a cesarean will be performed before the onset of labor—or even before the pregnancy has reached full term, if either the mother or the baby becomes endangered by bleeding.

Things You Need for Your New Arrival

Sorting though all the baby supplies in stores and catalogs can be overwhelming. This list, compiled from the advice of many parents, includes the items that most moms and dads have found truly useful. You can keep expenses down by postponing many purchases until you have had some hands-on experience with your baby. I could have used this advice years ago! When I was pregnant with Alexander, I found a very cute electric swing (that took up a lot of space) and insisted on buying it immediately. After his birth, we tried it once, he screamed, we tried it again, certain that he would love it. He didn't. He hated it, and he never sat in it again. He much preferred a small, vibrating chair that we carried from room to room with us. I ended up giving away the swing. If I had waited before buying, we could have tried it out in the store.

You might also borrow some items from friends or family members. Some things should not be borrowed or should be borrowed only with caution; in the following pages, I will explain which items this advice applies to.

Don't worry if your baby happens to arrive before you have all the baby things in place for her. She won't mind a bit!

Do You Need Two of Everything?

If you are pregnant with twins, it is not necessary to buy two of everything. Just as with one baby, you don't yet know what each child is like. You don't want to buy two swings, for example, if you don't know whether either baby will like swinging. If you find that both children love a vibrating bouncy chair, buy a second one when you need it—after they are born. You do, however, absolutely need two car seats. I suggest that parents of twins consider buying car seats that snap in and out of a double stroller base. This allows for easy transfer of the babies without waking them.

If you have identical twins, you may want to buy different-colored clothing for each baby to help tell them apart. You also want to consider whether the twins will share a room or have separate rooms. Often, one baby is a better sleeper than the other.

Here is my list of essentials for parents of twins:

- One twin breastfeeding pillow or two regular pillows
- Two baby packs or slings (one for each parent)
- Backpack diaper bag (so both your hands are free)
- Double stroller with two snap-in car seats
- One or two bouncy seats
- Two high chairs, for after the babies are about six months old
- One crib for the first three months, and two for after that
- Multiple changing stations (especially if you have a two-story house)
- High-quality electric double breast pump
- Bottle-propping pillow
- Extra bottles and nipples
- Preemie diapers bought well before the due date, just in case

Is a Hand-Me-Down Crib a Good Choice?

Many parents-to-be are lovingly given the family heirloom crib or have a friend who offers to lend them a crib that is no longer needed. Before you accept an offer of a crib, keep in mind the Consumer Product Safety Commission has set the following safety standards for cribs:

- The bars must not be more than 2⅜ inches (6 cm) apart.
- There must be no cracks in the wood.
- You'll want to purchase a new mattress if the previous one is more than five years old.
- The mattress level should be adjustable.
- The rail should be at least 22 inches (56 cm) above the top of the mattress, when the mattress is set at its highest level, and covered with plastic.
- There should be steel stabilizer bars.
- The side that drops must lock firmly into place.
- The mattress should fit snugly, with no more than two adult finger-widths between the crib and mattress.
- The mattress should have a sturdy, nonremovable, waterproof covering.

All new cribs sold in the United States should meet these standards. For more information on crib safety, or to check on a particular model, see the website of the Consumer Product Safety Commission, www.cpsc.gov.

THE BABY'S BED

You have plenty of choices about where your baby sleeps (or where you *try* to get your baby to sleep!). Whatever type of bed you choose, make sure that the item meets the safety standards that I outline on page 200.

Crib. Many parents lend or give away outgrown cribs. A crib should be borrowed carefully, however, especially if it is older. Be sure that the mattress has an intact, waterproof covering, or buy a new mattress. Check the crib against the safety standards listed on page 200. If the rails aren't covered with plastic, make sure that the finish is nontoxic.

My suggestion for twins is the same as for one baby—"easy access." Select the sleeping arrangement that allows you to tend to your babies as easily as possible so that you can return to sleep. When they are infants, it is easiest (and comforting to them) to have the babies sleep together in one crib. Many parents keep the crib in their bedroom for the first couple of months, and then move the babies into a shared crib in another room. Some children sleep well in the same crib until they move to regular beds but most eventually begin to wake one another up. At some point, you will want to have a second crib.

Bassinet or cradle. These are more portable than standard cribs and take up less space in the house. A bassinet usually has wheels, so you can keep it near your bedside during the night and move it around during the day. You'll want to be sure it has a sturdy, stable base. The advantage of a cradle, of course, is that it rocks. A cradle or bassinet should be used only until the baby can push himself up onto his knees or into a sitting position.

Three-sided sleeper. This specialized bassinet is open on one side and attaches to the side of an adult bed. A three-sided sleeper lets you keep your baby in a separate bed but within your reach at night. This arrangement is especially helpful in the early months, when you will be feeding the baby several times a night.

Portable crib-playpen. Most parents today rely on gates for confining their babies at home, but a portable crib-playpen is still very useful as a safe and clean place for a young baby to sleep and play, especially when the family is traveling (this is usually what you get, in fact, if you ask for a portable crib in a hotel). Today's models have more features than old-fashioned playpens did. Each can function as a crib, with a mattress that can be raised (for a newborn) or lowered. A removable changing table includes space for diapers, cloths, clothing, and other sundries. When the changing table is attached, the other side of the playpen can be used as a bassinet.

We used our portable crib-playpen all the time when Alexander was a baby. During the day, he napped in his crib in his own room, but during the night, he slept in our room. We set up the portable crib-playpen at the foot of our bed with the changing table in place. At night, Alexander could either stay in bed with us or settle in the bassinet. We never had to walk more than 5 feet (1.5 m) in the middle of the night.

BED LINENS

First, here's what you don't need:

- *Pillows.* These are often packaged with other crib linens. They are for decoration only; don't leave them in the crib with the baby.

- *Thick quilts or blankets.* If you are given these, use them on the floor for the baby to lie on or in the car as a warm covering, or just drape them decoratively over a chair. They shouldn't be used in the baby's bed.

Here is what I recommend getting:

- *Two or three fitted sheets.* Regular woven cotton is soft and cool; flannel is nice for cold weather. A fitted sheet should have at least 2 inches (5 cm) of fabric beneath the mattress so that the sheet can't slip off and entangle the baby.
- *One quilted mattress pad,* to go over the mattress.
- *Two felt-covered rubber sheets,* to lay over the mattress pad. Having two allows you to change the bedding without having to wait until a load of laundry is done.
- *Two or three light blankets.* Layering is the best way to keep baby warm. Avoid fringes or long, loose threads.

MOBILE

To entertain the baby when she wakes, you can hang one of these from the ceiling above her bed or attach it to the side of the crib. The Smith-Kettlewell Eye Research Institute of San Francisco says that objects that are pleasing to your own eyes will be pleasing to your baby's, so don't assume that a baby's mobile must be only black and white.

CHANGING PLACE

You can purchase a table made for diaper changing or use any other secure, flat surface with a washable pad on top. A dresser usually works well. You'll want the top to be at a comfortable height so that you don't need to lean down too far. It's nice, too, to have storage space for diapers and other things and an area to keep some supplies within easy reach. You don't need a strap to hold the baby in place; with or without a strap, you should always keep one hand on the baby at changing time.

Tori's Tip: Be Good to Yourself

You don't need to only use cloth diapers and a diaper service to be environmentally friendly. There are many options of nature-friendly disposable diapers that fit into a variety of needs and price ranges.

DIAPER CONTAINER

These are designed for either disposable or cloth diapers. If you will be using a diaper service, the service will provide the container (not all communities have a diaper service). If you are using disposable diapers, you can choose from containers in a variety of styles, some with high-tech bagging systems and none very expensive. All tend to be more convenient and less smelly than a regular trash can.

ELECTRONIC BABY MONITOR

This allows you to listen to and/or watch the baby while you are in a distant room. With a monitor, parents can feel more comfortable about doing things in other areas of the home. Because monitors operate within a certain radio frequency band, they run the risk of picking up signals from other electronic devices such as fluorescent lights or even a neighbor's phone. For this reason, some parents in more populated areas feel that a monitor is not worth the trouble. My husband and I once woke up to a very distressed child's cry of "Mommy!" and ran upstairs to tend to Alexander. Lo and behold, he was sound asleep! We then heard the crying coming from the kitchen. We were bewildered until we realized that the monitor in the kitchen was picking up the voice of a neighbor's child!

If you do decide to use a baby monitor, look for portability, ease of use, and a frequency that will not interfere with other wireless devices in your home.

BABY TUB

Some tubs stand alone; others fit into a bathtub or sink. Easy draining and portability are important features. You might instead buy (for about eight dollars) a foam pad that fits into a sink. Until about eight months of age, Alexander had all his baths in the kitchen sink. This was easy on my back, and we had a lot of fun splashing in the kitchen.

TUB SEAT

Once the baby is able to sit up, you can keep him from tipping with a restraint that sticks to the tub with suction cups. You can't rely on one of these, though; you must stay with the baby at all times when he is in the tub. Since you won't need a tub seat until the baby is about six months old, you can put off purchasing it until after he is born.

VIBRATING BOUNCY CHAIR

This is a small, inexpensive reclined seat that can be carried from room to room and that provides the options of a mild vibration and music. Whether asleep or awake, Alexander was often happy in one of these.

SWING

It can be small and simple or very elaborate with music and variable speeds. Your baby may or may not like swinging, so consider this before buying. This may be something to borrow, or wait until later to purchase.

STROLLER

Strollers come in many sizes and styles. Some versions are quite simple, and other, larger models have features almost like those on a luxury car! Visit stores to see which type and model best suit your needs. If money is no object, you may be tempted to go for the luxury, but a midrange model is probably your best bet. Before settling on one, look for the Juvenile Products Manufacturers Association (JPMA) certification.

These are some features you may want to consider:

Attachable infant car seat. Some strollers come with a car seat, and others allow you to snap in a car seat purchased separately. If you are also buying a car seat, make sure it will work with the stroller. These strollers tend to be large. An alternative is a stroller frame, which has no seat at all until you snap a car seat into it.

Reclining seat. The stroller may instantly convert to a carriage for a young baby, or recline for a napping older child.

Sun and rain shields. These can be bought separately.

Weight and portability. If you will frequently carry the stroller in the car, you'll want a model that is light and easy to fold.

Maneuverability. Most strollers now have nonfixed wheels for easy maneuverability.

Handle height. Make sure the handle is at the right height for you. Sometimes the height is adjustable.

Storage space. There may be a basket underneath and mesh sacks attached.

You may want to consider one of these special strollers:

Umbrella stroller. This lightweight, inexpensive type folds very easily and so is especially handy for traveling. Because the seat doesn't recline, however, an umbrella stroller can be used only after the baby is sitting up, and it is generally recommended for children at least one year old.

Jogging stroller. This kind of stroller has large wheels that provide a smooth ride on different types of terrain. A jogging stroller is a must if you want to push your baby along on runs or hikes. This stroller can't easily be carried in a car, so many families who use a jogging stroller also have a smaller, collapsable stroller.

Twin or double stroller. If you have twins or two children very close in age, you can choose between front-to-back and side-by-side seating. Side-by-side strollers seem to be more popular, perhaps because children usually like sitting side by side. Most of these strollers will fit through a 30-inch (76 cm) door, but you may want to measure the stroller before purchasing it.

CARRIAGE OR PRAM

When mothers primarily walked with their babies from home, these conveyances were quite popular. Today they are less so, but they can still be nice for neighborhood walking. A carriage (or a reclining stroller) can also be used at home as a portable bed.

Designed for young infants, a carriage is no longer useful when the baby is sitting up.

CAR SEAT

This is required by law whenever a baby rides in a car. You can choose from two types, one just for infancy, and the other for children from birth to 40 pounds (18 kg).

Infant car seat. This is suitable for babies up to 30 pounds (13.6 kg), depending on the model. With every model, the baby sits facing the rear of the car with a base that can be left in the car. The seat then snaps into and out of the base. The main advantages of this type of seat are that it is small, it can be removed with the baby in it, and it can be set on the ground or snapped into a stroller. Parents can easily transfer a sleeping baby into or out of the car without waking her. Infant car seats sometimes come as part of a stroller "system"; they can also be used with a stroller frame (page 205).

Convertible infant-toddler car seat. These larger seats can be used from infancy up to 40 pounds (18 kg). While the baby is very small, you'll need to surround him with a head support (you can buy one or use a rolled towel), as the seat will be much larger than he is. The seat is used rear facing until the baby is at least two years old and weighs at least 30 pounds (13.6 kg). In fact, it is best for children to ride rear facing until they are the greatest height or weight (usually 30 pounds [13.6 kg] or more) specified by the manufacturer. You can then turn the seat face forward and continue to use it until your child weights 40 pounds (18 kg), at which point he'll graduate to a booster seat. All convertible car seats should have a harness that fastens at five points; do not use one that does not have a five-point restraint system. Look for a seat that is easy to install and to adjust and is comfortable for the baby.

BABY CARRIER

A baby sling or pack lets you keep your baby close to you and happy while your hands are free. Select a carrier that is washable, easy to adjust, and comfortable for you. I recommend trying on different ones in a store and putting your purse in them to see how they feel on your back. When Alexander was a baby, I preferred a sling, and Ray liked a soft front pack, so we bought both.

When your baby is about six months old, you can move her to a backpack with a frame. It will work well until your child becomes too heavy to carry.

DIAPER BAG

Thank goodness these have become more fashionable! Every major handbag designer is making an expensive diaper bag these days, but you can also find inexpensive bags that look just as attractive as the designer ones. Most diaper bags are large handbags or shoulder bags; some are fashionable backpacks. Look for a bag with multiple compartments, a place for a bottle, a plastic lining, and a zipper closing. Some bags also come with slim changing pads.

BREASTFEEDING SUPPLIES

If you will be with your baby at all times, the only special feeding supplies you may need are nursing bras, with flaps that lower for easy access to the breast; modified lanolin in case your nipples get sore (page 352); and either washable or disposable nursing pads, which go in your bra to absorb leaking milk.

Exclusively breastfeeding is a wonderful gift you can give to your baby. But that doesn't mean that you shouldn't be able to spend some time with yourself and have a loved one feed your baby. Or, perhaps you are heading back to work and want to be able to feed your baby your breast milk. There are several different types of breast pumps you can choose from. Let's start from the simplest.

What Is So Great About Breastfeeding?

The American Academy of Pediatrics (AAP) says that it is healthiest for babies to be exclusively breastfed for the first six months of life and to continue to be breastfed at least until the first birthday. AAP research confirms that babies who are breastfed enjoy several benefits:

- They receive all the nutrients (protein, fat, carbohydrates, vitamins, and minerals) that are necessary for growth for the first six months of life.
- They have less stomach upset and gas than do formula-fed babies, because breast milk is easily digested.
- They receive antibodies from their mothers against a variety of illnesses.
- They have fewer respiratory illnesses and ear infections and less diarrhea than formula-fed babies have.
- They may be provided some protection against chronic diseases, including asthma, insulin-dependent diabetes, ulcerative colitis, and some childhood forms of leukemia and lymphoma.
- They may be provided some protection against Sudden Infant Death Syndrome (SIDS).

Manual Pump

These are certainly the smallest, least expensive, and most portable of all the options. They are cost effective and straightforward to use. But they are a bit more work. They work by pressing with either one or both hands to express your milk.

Portable Electric Pump

This is the most commonly used pump for women who are going back to work or who would like to be able to efficiently pump at home for an extra supply of milk. These generally come with a carrying case and the option to use a battery when necessary. They often contain a cooling storage container for times when you are not able to refrigerate your milk right away.

Hospital-Grade Electric Pump

You can rent a hospital grade electric pump, which works quickly and powerfully to pump both breasts at the same time. These pumps are not portable and are rather expensive, so you would likely not purchase one. They are, however, readily available to rent. In my experience, they are more likely used in a hospital setting for babies who may need to stay a bit longer, are premature, or who are having some difficulties breast-feeding. There is often a "nursing" room where new moms can pump in private when they are unable to nurse their babies directly.

I chose the Medela Pump in Style. Though fairly expensive (over $300 in 2017), this model worked well for me. It is lightweight, compact, and easy to carry in its attractive case. I have since lent my pump to four or five friends, leaving out the plastic attachments, which are not to be used by more than one mother. Because a high-quality pump, consumer- or hospital-grade, is merely a motor, it's fine to lend or borrow it. New attachments should be available wherever the pump was originally purchased or rented.

If your family income qualifies, you may be able to borrow a pump through the Supplemental Nutrition Program for Women, Infants, and Children (WIC). Your childbirth educator or a staff member at your hospital or birth center can probably refer you to a source for breast pumps. If not, contact one of the organizations listed under "Sources for Breastfeeding Support and Breast Pumps" (page 211).

Sources for Breastfeeding Support and Breast Pumps

Your hospital or birth center may offer breastfeeding classes, breast pumps for sale or rent, and the services of a lactation consultant. Other organizations also provide breastfeeding resources:

- The International Lactation Consultant Association provides referrals of local lactation consultants. Call 919-861-5577, visit the website at www.ilca.org, or send an e-mail message to info@ilca.org.
- La Leche League provides group meetings and mother-to-mother breastfeeding advice. Call 800-LA LECHE, visit the website at llli.org, or check the white pages of your phone book.
- Some other mothers' groups, such as Mothers of Twins (www.nomotc.org) and Nursing Mothers Counsel (www.nursingmothers.org), provide breastfeeding support as well.
- In some cities, lactation consultants provide breastfeeding counseling in stores where you can also get nursing bras, pumps, and other supplies.
- Medela, the largest manufacturer of breast pumps, provides referrals to lactation consultants and pump-rental stations at 800-TELL-YOU and information about its products at 800-435-8316 and on its website, www.medela.com.

You may also want to buy some supplies for storing your milk. Some companies sell breast-milk storage "systems" that include bottles, nipples, and plastic bags for freezing breast milk. The advantage of bags over rigid containers is that they take up less space in your freezer. For various reasons, you might breastfeed your baby only part-time or for a short time. In this case, remember that any amount of breast milk your baby receives can improve his health, by providing immunological substances and nutrients that are unavailable in formula.

BOTTLE-FEEDING SUPPLIES

You'll need supplies for bottle feeding if you intend to go back to work and pump your milk, if you plan to feed formula part-time, or if your baby will be entirely formula fed.

Not too many years ago, babies' bottles were mostly uniform. Today, there are many shapes, styles, and sizes, and manufacturers claim each model to be better, improved, or more natural. A good bottle is easy to fill, easy to store, and easy to wash. All should be BPA-free and top rack dishwasher safe. Some models come with disposable plastic liners designed to help keep air out so that the baby swallows less air. Most bottles can be washed either by hand or in the dishwasher; check the label to be sure.

As with bottles, there are many types of nipples on the market. You can choose from rubber or silicone, in a variety of lengths and shapes. Rubber nipples should be washed by hand; silicone nipples can go in the dishwasher. Some nipples fit only certain bottles, and vice versa. You can ask your baby's doctor which type he or she recommends, or start with samples from your hospital or birth center.

Since you and your baby may find that you prefer one type of bottle and nipple to another, you may want to start with one bottle and nipple for each of two or three types. I made the mistake of buying an entire "system" before Alexander was born. When I started using it, I found that Alexander didn't like it at all.

Once you have settled on a type, the number of bottles and nipples you'll need will vary depending on whether you are formula feeding or breastfeeding and, if you're breastfeeding, how often your baby will be taking your pumped milk. In any case, I suggest starting with two to four 8-ounce bottles, two to four 4-ounce bottles, and four nipples. If you are breastfeeding, you won't need these until the time you may want to introduce a bottle, when your baby is about three weeks old. I found that this made it easier for me to spend a little time away from Alexander and allowed Ray to feed him my breast milk.

Especially if you will be washing bottles entirely by hand, I recommend buying a bottle brush to make the job easier. Bottle brushes are available in the baby sections of most supermarkets.

A bottle warmer is by no means necessary, but it is convenient. Alternatively, you can warm your bottle in a cup of water from the sink.

YOUR BABY'S WARDROBE

The initial size for baby clothes is 0 to 3 months; the next is 3 to 6 months. Because babies grow fast, you won't want to spend a lot on clothing in these sizes. Even though Alexander was only 6 pounds, 12 ounces (3 kg), at birth, he grew so quickly that we barely used the size 0 to 3-months outfits. Many babies fit into size 3 to 6-months clothes at birth!

Clothing in these sizes gets so little use that hand-me-downs are usually in excellent condition. Accept any offers from friends or family members. Secondhand stores and yard sales are other good options. When you buy any baby clothes, keep in mind how big your baby is likely to be in the upcoming seasons.

For a premature baby, you may want clothing even smaller than size 0 to 3-months. Preemie-size clothes can be hard to find, but the staff at the hospital where the baby was born may be able to tell you where you can purchase some.

Here are the types of clothes you're likely to want for your baby:

Snap-bottom body shirts. You'll probably need four to six. The baby undershirt has been mostly replaced by these one-piece undershirts, because they don't ride up, keeping the baby's tummy warm. On a warm day, your little one may wear nothing else besides a diaper. In cooler weather, you can add a pair of pull-up pants and a shirt or sweater.

Gowns. I like the sacklike gowns with elastic at the bottom. Especially during the night, diaper changes are easier when you don't have to fuss with snaps. You'll probably want two to four gowns.

Booties or socks. Newborns' little feet always seem to get cold. Socks tend to stay on better than booties, but *either* type is fine. You'll want to have plenty on hand—say, six to eight pairs—because they are tiny and thus can easily get lost in the wash.

Pull-on stretch pants. You'll need four to six. These are good for daytime dressing with snap-bottom shirts and sweaters. You'll need four to six pairs of pants.

One-piece suits. These are used as sleepwear for older babies, and many newborns wear them day and *night.* They can be found in light cotton knits, cozy fleece, and a variety of other fabrics. Footed suits eliminate the need for socks. Suits without feet are good for warmer days and for when the baby begins to play with her feet.

Hooded terry-cloth towels. These are wonderful for keeping your baby's head and body warm and covered after a bath. It's nice to have two.

Sweaters or jackets. These may not get much use when your baby is a newborn, but after he is three months old or so, you will probably take him out more. Two lightweight sweaters or jackets for warmer weather and two heavier ones for chilly days are about all you'll need.

Hats. These are essential in cold weather. And when your baby is out in the sun, a sun hat is a must! It's nice to have an extra hat or two in case one is lost.

Snowsuit or bunting. One of these warm items is necessary if you are taking the baby out in winter weather. Be sure that a snowsuit is easy to take on and off. Because they have no sleeves, buntings, which are usually made of very warm fleece, are easier to use. Many buntings have divided legs so that you can put your little one in a stroller or car seat and buckle the strap between the baby's legs.

Receiving blanket. These thin, lightweight blankets are great for swaddling and for lightly covering the baby. They are also a handy cover-up for breastfeeding privacy. Three blankets will probably be enough.

DISPOSABLE DIAPERS

If you are planning to use disposable diapers, have one to two dozen on hand before your baby's birth, some in newborn size and some in size one. If you are giving birth in a hospital, you will probably go home with another stack. Don't buy a large quantity of any particular brand until you have tried two or more brands, because you may like one better than another. (Your preferred brand may not be the most expensive, either.) Once you know which works best for you—which type leaks the least, seems the most comfortable for the baby, and is the easiest to use—then buy in larger quantities. Disposable diapers are expensive, so you'll want to get the best for the money.

If you *would* like to take a more ecological approach to diapering but don't want to use cloth, check out the "natural" disposables, which contain less plastic and absorbent gel or even no gel or plastic at all. These diapers are available at most baby-supply stores and online.

Even if you will mainly be using cloth diapers, you may want to have some disposables on hand. Many people who use cloth diapers find that disposables are more convenient at night or when the family is traveling.

CLOTH DIAPERS

A diaper service will provide you with these, in the appropriate size, along with a diaper pail (sign up for a service now if you haven't already). If you will be washing your own diapers, I recommend getting four to five dozen prefolded ones.

Even if you're using disposables, you may want a supply of clean cloth diapers to place over your shoulder as burp cloths. They will save your nice blouses from mommy spots!

DIAPER WRAPS AND COVERS

A necessity if you are using cloth diapers, wraps and other covers come in various styles, fabrics, and sizes. Some covers are waterproof; others are very absorbent. You can choose from elasticized ones that pull on and those with Velcro-type fasteners. Many covers allow for diapering without pins or other fasteners, although you may want to have a few diaper pins on hand for when a Velcro-type fastener isn't sticking well.

WIPES

For simplicity, you can clean the baby's bottom with a small washcloth and warm water. For convenience, though, you may want to use disposable wipes. Numerous brands are available, and the most expensive is not necessarily any better than a discount brand. I found that some brands were stronger and softer on the baby's skin than others. Because newborn skin is delicate, start with a brand with no perfumes or alcohol.

WIPE WARMER

I am a minimalist when it comes to baby stuff, but this item is on my must-have list. A wipe warmer is a small, heated container that holds a pack of disposable wipes and keeps them at a consistent warm temperature. We had a much happier baby when we touched Alexander's bottom at 3:00 A.M. with a warm wipe rather than a chilly one.

BURP CLOTHS

You'll want about a dozen cloths for keeping the baby's spit-up off your clothes. You can buy cloths marketed as burp cloths with cute designs on them, but prefolded cloth diapers work just as well. I suggest keeping one in your diaper bag, one in the car, and one in each room of the house.

HIGH CHAIR

You don't need to begin looking for one of these until the baby is able to sit up on her own, at about six months. By then, you will have a better idea of the kinds of products you like.

CHILDPROOFING SUPPLIES

Many items are available to protect your baby from dangers in and around your home. Useful safety supplies include drawer and cabinet latches, outlet plug covers, and stove knob covers. By the time your baby is six to eight months old, you will want to assess your home for safety and install some of these protective devices. Or you can hire a professional who will come into your home and childproof it for you.

SAFETY GATES

If you have a home with stairs or wish to restrict your baby to one area, you'll want to use one or more baby gates. They can be anything from a simple plastic barrier fit in the doorframe to a fully finished oak gate that swings open and latches shut.

MEDICAL SUPPLIES AND TOILETRIES

These are the supplies you are most likely to need for grooming your baby and caring for his health. All are available in drugstores; many supplies are available in grocery stores as well.

- *Infant acetaminophen*, for fever.
- *Sunscreen*, for use only after the first six months.
- *Calibrated dropper*, for administering medicine.
- *Bulb syringe (or similar suction device)*, for clearing a stuffy nose.
- *Baby nail clippers or scissors*.
- *Basic digital thermometer*, for taking the baby's temperature under their armpit or rectally (ear and forehead thermometers are not always accurate at a very young age). Ask your baby's doctor about how to do this, and see page 346. Never take your baby's temperature rectally unless instructed by your pediatrician!
- *Diaper-rash ointment*. I prefer Aquaphor, an ointment containing lanolin and mineral oil.
- *Petroleum jelly or Aquaphor*, to protect a newly circumcised penis from urine.
- *Baby brush and comb*.
- *Pedialyte or Ricelyte*, for hydration in case the baby has vomiting or diarrhea (only if instructed to use by your pediatrician).

- *Activated charcoal*, to treat poisoning. Use it only on the recommendation of a physician or poison-control center (the national poison-control telephone number is 800-222-1222). The American Academy of Pediatrics no longer recommends that syrup of ipecac be used in the home to induce vomiting.
- *Baby bath wash or gentle glycerin soap.* Use this sparingly, or not at all if your baby has sensitive skin. Babies become quite clean with water alone!
- *Baby shampoo.* Or use baby bath wash instead.

Lotions and powders are not necessary for your baby; they can be irritating to delicate skin. With all toiletries, less is almost always best for a baby.

Ask Tori, R.N.

IDENTICAL TWINS

Dear Tori,

I had twin girls four years ago. When I was pregnant, I was told they were in separate sacs and therefore not identical. Once they were born, the doctor said they might be identical, because they had the same blood type. They look very much alike, and I am asked all the time if they are identical. Is there any way to know for sure whether they are identical or fraternal?

—Lisa, Maine

Dear Lisa,

Identical twins occur when one egg divides into two, so that the babies have the same genetic makeup. Fraternal twins occur when two separate eggs are fertilized.

Like fraternal twins, identical twins normally have two separate amniotic sacs. It is extremely rare for these twins to share one sac, and dangerous, too, since the babies' umbilical cords could get entangled during the pregnancy.

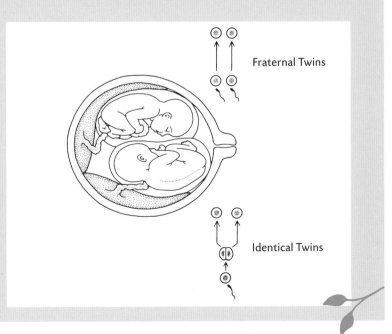

Fraternal Twins

Identical Twins

Your girls could indeed be identical, especially if they look a great deal alike. The fact that they have the same blood type isn't a clear indication, as it is quite common for siblings within any family to have the same blood type. The only way to know for certain is to have the girls genetically tested. Their doctor should be able to help you find out how to do this and the costs involved.

GENITAL HERPES

Tori,

I am 30 weeks pregnant, and I've noticed little pimples that erupted just outside my vagina and that are starting to itch. I have had genital herpes before (although I haven't had an outbreak for a couple of years), and I believe it may be back. Should I be concerned, should I take anything, or should I just wait for the eruption to go away? I know this could be a problem if I were about to go into labor, but that isn't the case. What are the concerns at this point in my pregnancy ?

—Maria, Pennsylvania

Dear Maria,

Any time you experience some new or unusual physical condition, whether you are pregnant or not, it is important to have a doctor or another medical practitioner check it out. Your symptoms may indicate genital herpes or another condition that should be treated. Let your practitioner know that you have had genital herpes outbreaks before.

Genital herpes is a sexually transmitted infection caused by the herpes simplex virus. Between 20 and 25 percent of pregnant women have genital herpes. Women who have outbreaks at birth risk transmitting the virus to their babies, for whom the infection could be life threatening. In this case, a cesarean section is the safest way to deliver.

If you have a genital herpes lesion, it will not cause any problem as long as it heals within the next couple of weeks. Your doctor or midwife should discuss treatment options with you. Antiviral medications are considered safe to use in pregnancy and some women with more frequent outbreaks take medication daily. There are new treatment options coming out all the time.

FIFTH DISEASE

Tori,

Help! My mother was recently exposed to fifth disease. I'm seven months pregnant, and I have been advised to stay away from my mother. I had never heard of fifth disease before; it's not even mentioned in the books I've looked at. What are the symptoms, how dangerous could it be to my baby, and what should I do now ?

—Alexis, West Virginia

Alexis,

Fifth disease, caused by a parvovirus, is so called because it is the fifth in a group of six childhood diseases that cause rash and fever. The symptoms of rash and fever are generally mild and frequently go unnoticed. It is uncommon to develop fifth disease during pregnancy. Most women are in fact immune, having been infected as children without being aware of the infection.

Very rarely, infection with fifth disease during pregnancy increases the risk of an early miscarriage or a rare form of fetal anemia. It is best to follow your practitioner's advice in your situation, but you and your baby are likely to be completely unaffected.

VAGINAL BIRTH AFTER CESAREANS

Dear Tori,

My mother, who is now in her sixties, delivered all of her children by cesarean section. Now my doctor says it is safe for me to have my baby vaginally, even though I have had one C-section. My mother says vaginal birth would be dangerous for me. I am confused.

—Alicia, Georgia

Dear Alicia,

Cesarean sections are performed differently today from when your mother had her babies. The surgery requires two incisions, one through the mother's skin and the other in the mother's uterus. The skin incision, which has no effect on future deliveries, is today usually made horizontally, at or below the pubic hair line (this is called a *bikini incision)*. Your mom probably had a larger, vertical skin incision along her entire abdomen. The more important incision, though, is the one made in the uterus. When your mom had her cesareans, her uterine incision was probably also vertical, or *classical*. Today, cesareans are performed with horizontal uterine and skin incisions. A horizontal uterine incision is called *low transverse*.

Because uterine fibers form in a striated, vertical fashion, a vertical uterine scar tends to be weak. If, during a subsequent labor, the uterus were to contract intensely along the scar, the uterus might tear open, a condition that would be life threatening for both mom and baby. For this reason, women of your mother's generation were advised against going through labor after having had a cesarean section.

A horizontal uterine incision forms a much stronger scar. As several studies confirmed in the early 1990s, this type of incision makes it safe to attempt a vaginal birth after cesarean (VBAC) with a second pregnancy. More recent studies have found a small risk—1 in 200 to 400 chance—of the uterus's tearing during VBAC with a horizontal incision. (The risk is much greater after multiple cesareans.) Because of these latter findings, the trend toward repeat cesarean sections has increased in recent years. Yet many women still choose VBAC, and 70 percent of those who do elect this type of delivery succeed in delivering vaginally.

VBAC is essentially no different from any other vaginal birth, but the medical staff monitors the mother's labor carefully to be sure the scar doesn't separate. In the rare case of scar separation, a repeat cesarean is performed.

Although VBAC continues to carry lower risks of infection and postpartum complications than does cesarean birth, some physicians refuse to attend a VBAC. If you would prefer a VBAC to a repeat cesarean, I suggest looking for a physician who may be willing to assist you, depending on your obstetrical history.

You have a greater chance of a successful VBAC if all the following conditions apply:

- Your pregnancy is progressing normally, and you have no medical complications.
- Your labor begins spontaneously between 37 and 40 weeks' gestation.
- The reason for the prior cesarean (such as a breech baby) is not a factor this time.
- You are younger than 40.
- Your baby is no bigger than 8½ pounds (3.9 kg) when labor begins.
- You have delivered vaginally before.
- You have had only one prior cesarean, with a low transverse uterine incision.

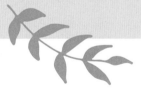

DAD'S CORNER

There are a few simple things you can do to help get ready for the baby. For example, you could create something that you can leave behind when you are away at work or traveling, something that says you are thinking about your partner and your new baby:

Make a music playlist for your spouse. You might include only soft music, perhaps for her to practice relaxing to, or just combine her favorite tunes.

Make a playlist of classical music or simple songs that you love. Use it to introduce your baby to music.

Take a clear picture of your face and another of your partner's face, and make several prints of each. After your baby is born, you can place one in the crib and one or two in play areas at baby's eye level. Your picture will be especially appreciated if you travel a great deal or serve in the military.

Mom is not the only one who will be carrying the baby once she is born, so **consider choosing a baby carrier** for your own use. There are many types of carriers, and chances are, you will prefer one that is different from the one your partner selects. It's much easier to go for a walk or soothe a fussy baby if you don't have to be continually adjusting straps.

Use your excess energy to **organize things for the new baby.** Some men (not to make any assumptions) get a little wound up as their partners' pregnancies move into the last trimester. If you are itching to do something, ask friends and relatives if they will be willing to help out after the birth. You might draw up a schedule of who will help with the plants, pets, cooking, and so on. You might even get together with other dads-to-be and fix up each family's nursery in turn. One group of friends who did this reported a great sense of accomplishment at having talked and worked together, all in a relaxed atmosphere.

Treat Her Well. Prepare an entire dinner for her: Create the menu, shop, cook, serve, and clean up afterward. If you are the chief cook in the household, make this a truly special meal. If you are not very skilled in the kitchen, don't worry—a not-so-gourmet meal can still be great fun and will make for a wonderful memory.

Tori's Tip:
Beware the "Madonna Phenomenon"

If you have recently glanced through women's magazines, how-to books on fathering, and news articles about celebrity moms, you might conclude that new mothers are treated like royalty, or at least the mothers of royalty. By these accounts, new mothers glow, parents and in-laws dote, partners are awed, and girlfriends constantly stream in to help with the house, the kids, and the shopping. Communities provide daily casseroles and comfy slippers. All this is supposed to happen because mothers bring the miracle of new life. But does it really happen?

Ask your mother or grandmother what things were like when she had her babies. Was she treated like a queen? How was it for your sister or your friend? Was she pampered, protected, and served hand and foot? Maybe, or maybe not.

When I ask new mothers if they have gotten the queen-bee treatment, most say, "The what?" Of course, some respond, "My husband is the best ever!" or "I rely a lot on my sister; she comes by every day." Many women, though, feel that when people come to visit the new baby, it is just simply exhausting. Some mothers say that people were helpful with the first baby, but not the second. One mom told me that her co-workers' only response to her having a baby was to be more demanding immediately before she took maternity leave.

The image of the Holy Madonna, a woman tenderly cradling a newborn, has been immortalized in everything from sculpture to holiday postage stamps. For rock-star-cum-diva Madonna, pregnancy and childbirth became a passage to mainstream acceptance. *That same* Madonna a saintly Madonna? The woman who in her early career was known as Boy Toy? The woman whose performance in Italy was censored by the pope? Yes, the very woman who, smoothly coifed and dressed in pastels, later appeared on the cover of Good Housekeeping magazine. Motherhood made her safe.

For very rich, royal, or famous women, labor and childbirth are a public event. For a movie star giving birth, the fanfare can be staggering. The public has happily followed the births of England's little Prince George and Princess Charlotte. However, when Prince William speaks of his mother, Princess Diana, we have come to understand that despite all of the celebrity excitement, she was bulimic and depressed. Finally, more and more women in the public eye have spoken openly about their struggles with this "Madonna phenomenon" and post partum depression. Brooke Shields, Gwyneth Paltrow, Chrissy Teigen, and Hayden Panettiere are just a few.

Sadly, people respond better to the image of motherhood than to mothers themselves. Few women can go through early motherhood with the assistance of two nannies, a night nurse, and a personal trainer, but we all deserve to be treated like a Madonna, honored and pampered for bringing forth life. The more practical assistance and moral support a woman receives, the happier and healthier both she and her infant will be.

I started noticing the fascination with the image of motherhood during my pregnancy with Alexander. As my belly grew, so did the smiles and gentle or nosy comments from strangers. When Alexander was a newborn, people peeked into his stroller and cooed. When he was 6 months old, they enjoyed the smiles and laughter he gave them in return. But when he was 18 months old and having a tantrum and running behind a store counter, I realized that my image as Madonna, and his as adored prince, had faded. It was clear to me then that the Madonna myth needed to be replaced by a deeper respect for the incredible challenges of motherhood and a greater appreciation for its rewards.

Are We There Yet?
YOUR EIGHTH MONTH: WEEKS 32 THROUGH 35

DURING THE SECOND TRIMESTER, you may have felt exceptionally good. Your morning sickness may have passed, you may have had more energy, and you were probably enjoying your pregnancy. Now that you are well into your third trimester, though, you may have noticed some new and less pleasant sensations. Your emotions may feel more intense. Impatience for your pregnancy to be over, excitement and nervousness about becoming a parent, and apprehension about your upcoming labor—all these emotions may be running through your head.

You may feel that your body, your emotions, or your life is out of your control. This feeling can be unsettling. Used to planning your day, your week, your life, and carrying out these plans, you may have planned your pregnancy and assumed it would go a certain way. Maybe it is much as you predicted, but maybe not. In many ways, pregnancy is unpredictable.

For years, I wished to be pregnant. I looked forward to pregnancy and imagined what it would be like. Soon after I got pregnant, I became extremely nauseated and fatigued and was unable to stay awake. In my third trimester, Alexander tucked his feet under my ribs, and I felt as though a shoehorn were stretching my bones. And I had thought pregnancy would be fun! For my best girlfriend, it *was* fun, although before she became pregnant, she was quite afraid of labor. During her pregnancy, she thought the sky was brighter and the flowers smelled sweeter. Neither of us could have predicted what pregnancy would be like for us, and neither of us could control the experience.

You can't control the emotional experience of pregnancy any more than you can control the physical. You and your spouse are going through a major transition as you prepare for your baby's birth. It is normal to have conflicting emotions and to feel anxious about the birth, parenting, finances, and a host of other issues in your own life. Try to give yourself a break. Slow down, rest, and play a little more. Honor what is happening within your body. Allow yourself to be emotional without needing to figure out why. Cry if you need to.

Accept your mate's changing emotions as well. Don't expect him to be as expressive as you. If he seems a little distant or uninvolved in the pregnancy, this doesn't mean he won't be happy and involved with the new baby.

Labor is no more predictable than pregnancy, and as you become a parent, you will find many other things that are out of your control—the first being your little baby's personality and temperament. Letting go of some desire for control may help you become a better and more relaxed mother and person in general.

WHAT'S HAPPENING WITH YOUR BABY?

You have probably noticed that your abdomen has grown quite dramatically since last month. For the next two months, your baby will be gaining "brown" fat and putting on weight. Brown fat is necessary for the survival of newborn humans and other mammals. This special type of fat helps the baby to maintain his body heat.

Your baby will weigh about 4 to 5 pounds (1.8 to 2.3 kg) by the end of this month. His physical features are well developed, although he is still very lean. His brain is functioning at a very high capacity, and the only parts of his body yet to fully mature are his lungs.

Since your baby is growing larger, he is likely to be settling down into one position. He is rapidly running out of room to turn somersaults and will most likely remain in a head-down (vertex) position.

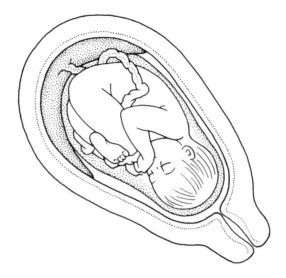

When a baby is head-down at birth, the skull stretches the cervix and molds to fit between the pelvic bones; the smaller, more flexible legs and torso can then pass easily.

If, instead, the baby is in a breech position, with his bottom or feet down, these parts of his body could deliver easily, but his head could become trapped in the uterus or behind the bones of your pelvis. To avoid this problem, your practitioner may attempt to perform an *external version*, a way of turning the baby into a head-down position. This is usually done in the 37th week.

With the guidance of an ultrasound machine, the practitioner applies a series of specific hand movements to your abdomen. Success depends on the position of the baby and the structure of the uterus, but in at least 50 percent of cases, the procedure works: The baby turns and stays in a vertex position. If external version doesn't work for you, your practitioner may feel it is safest to deliver the baby by cesarean section. For more on breech babies, see page 245.

WHAT'S HAPPENING WITH YOUR BODY?

As you near the end of pregnancy, you may notice more bodily changes. You may be experiencing more prelabor, or Braxton-Hicks, contractions. Your vaginal discharge may become thicker and whiter. As your body works very hard to provide oxygen and nutrients to your baby, you may fatigue easily and become quite sleepy during the day. Your increasing size may be starting to affect your mobility. And pregnancy may bring some novelty to your sex life.

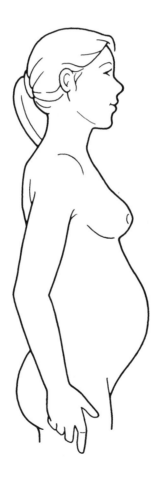

A Little More about Sex

I discussed lovemaking on 128 to 130, but concerns about sex tend to come up again about this time in pregnancy. Pregnancy brings an increased blood supply to the pelvic area, intensifying sensations, and for this reason, most women find lovemaking in the second and third trimesters very enjoyable. But in late pregnancy, a number of new concerns about sex may arise.

Your breasts have changed in preparation for feeding your baby. They have increased in size, and during sexual arousal, they or your nipples may enlarge even further. You may enjoy having your breasts fondled, or their tenderness may make stimulation uncomfortable and positioning important. You may leak colostrum (page 334) when your breasts are stimulated. For you and your partner, this may be arousing, or it may be unnerving. Know that this leakage is normal.

The size of the baby and your belly may make positioning for intercourse a challenge. You will probably find that lying on your side, getting on your hands and knees with your partner behind you, or getting on top of him will be the most comfortable.

Your baby will probably "drop" into your pelvis, or "engage," in the last couple of weeks of your pregnancy, although sometimes this happens only after labor begins. Once the baby drops, you may find that any increased pressure in your pelvic area and vagina is uncomfortable. Women sometimes ask, "How could there possibly be room for anything else in there?" Fathers may worry about the safety of mother and baby and so may hesitate to make sexual advances.

Hormones can cause changes in your vaginal lubrication. Most women experience an increase in secretions, but some notice a decrease. Dryness can cause irritation and make intercourse painful. A water-soluble lubricant such as AstroGlide or K-Y Jelly can solve this problem and is perfectly safe to use.

Pregnancy hormones make women more susceptible to vaginal yeast infections, which are itchy and sometimes painful. Oral medications are most effective, but they are not considered safe during pregnancy. A messy cream or suppository is the necessary treatment.

Many women find that during pregnancy, it is easier to achieve an orgasm. When you have an orgasm, the uterus contracts rhythmically. When you aren't pregnant, these contractions last from a few seconds to a few minutes. During pregnancy, they last longer and can be uncomfortable. This generally does not mean that the contractions are initiating labor prematurely. If, however, you are considered at risk for preterm labor, your doctor may give you instructions on limiting your sexual activity.

Sex has long been touted as a good "labor inducer." It would be great if induction were that easy. In the experience of many women I've talked with, the odds of initiating labor with intercourse, at term and with a partially softened and effaced cervix, is somewhere around 25 percent. And it probably isn't the contractions caused by orgasm that sometimes get things going; it is the prostaglandins in the partner's semen that seem to do the trick. So making love is an unreliable way to try to start labor—although it certainly can be fun!

It is sometimes hard for a woman, and her partner, to feel sexy in pregnancy. Her growing waistline constantly reminds her that she is going to be a mother. This may conflict with her view of herself as a sexual being. The enlarging belly may also remind Dad of the many responsibilities he will assume very soon. I was lucky to have a husband who loved my pregnant body, often more than I did, and so helped me feel sexy. If you don't feel sexy, though, that is just fine. If wearing only snuggly, flannel pajamas feels right, then that's what you should wear. Remember, you are the same woman you were before you were pregnant. Your blossoming body doesn't change that.

Common Discomforts

At this time in pregnancy, many women experience one or more of several conditions. Besides trying the suggestions listed here, you can take comfort in knowing that your discomfort will end shortly!

DISTURBED SLEEP

Your sleep at night is much less likely to be as continuous or deep as before you were pregnant. Not only may you have to get up to go to the bathroom several times during the night, but it may also be difficult to find and stay in a comfortable position.

The side-lying position helps take pressure off your lower back. Try using a pillow to support your abdomen and another one to support your upper leg. Also try leaning against a bunched-up pillow or rolled-up blanket placed at the small of your back. This can help take some of the pressure off the hip you're lying on.

Lying on your side also takes pressure off the large blood vessels that carry blood from your legs and feet back to your heart. Blood flow to your heart is slightly better when you are lying on your left side. Many books lead you to believe that you should *always* lie on your left side, but this is unnecessary. After all, our species survived a long time before we knew to do this!

LEAKING URINE

In my eighth month of pregnancy, I developed a cold and could not stop coughing. I was also very sore from Alexander's kicking and stretching my ribs. At the end of the day, while I was getting undressed to take a shower and Ray was brushing his teeth, I went into a coughing fit. Suddenly—I couldn't help it—I coughed and peed on the floor at the same time. I couldn't believe it! I didn't know whether to laugh or cry. Then both of us had a good laugh.

The increased pressure of your uterus and growing baby on your bladder may cause you, too, to leak urine from time to time. This may happen most often when you laugh, cough, or sneeze.

If you're experiencing occasional incontinence, be sure to pee whenever you have the urge—although I can't imagine how you could hold your urine for long. Do Kegel exercises (page 150); they can help decrease urine leaks by strengthening your perineal and vaginal muscles. You may also want to wear a panty liner, just in case. Finally, be sure to let your doctor or midwife know about the problem, since urinary incontinence can be a sign of a bladder infection.

SKIN CHANGES

As your skin stretches during late pregnancy, it may tend to become dry and itchy, especially on the abdomen and breasts. Scratching tends to make the problem worse. Instead, keep your skin well moisturized with lotion. If you are really uncomfortable, you can try an over-the-counter anti-itch cream containing 1 percent hydrocortisone.

If your baby has a sudden growth spurt, you may notice reddish or whitish streaks on your abdomen, especially if you are fair-skinned. Some women, particularly those with twins or triplets or who have gained weight rapidly, get these stretch marks on their breasts, hips, buttocks, or thighs. You many already have such marks from a period of fast growth during adolescence. Unfortunately, stretch marks can't be prevented, and there is no proven treatment for them. Because they develop from deep within the connective tissue underneath the skin, no miracle creams or ointments will make them magically vanish. Often, however, they will fade slowly after birth.

> ### Tori's Tip: Take a Break!
> It is extremely helpful to take a nap—even for 15 minutes—or at least to put your feet up at some point during the day.

SWOLLEN LEGS AND FEET

Your increased blood volume and pressure from the growing baby and uterus makes it harder for blood and fluid to flow back up from your lower legs. If you are on your feet quite a bit during the day, you will notice swelling (edema) in your feet, ankles, and legs, especially at the end of the day. Although edema can be a sign of preeclampsia (page 194), it is usually just a normal discomfort of late pregnancy.

Here are some ways to help relieve the discomfort of swollen feet and legs:

- Avoid standing for long periods.
- Don't sit with your legs crossed. This position can increase the pooling of fluid in your lower legs.

- Elevate your legs whenever you can. When sitting, rest them on another chair, an ottoman, or a stool. When lying down, raise your legs and feet on a pillow or two, especially if you find yourself sleeping on your back.
- Exercise regularly to keep your leg muscles moving. This will help improve your overall blood flow.
- Go swimming. Even standing or walking in a pool provides hydrostatic pressure to help move some of the fluid that has pooled in the legs, feet, and ankles.
- Use compression stockings, or support hose, to help improve the return of blood to your heart and thus decrease the fluid in your legs. Your doctor or midwife may be able to recommend a good brand.

During the last couple of weeks of my pregnancy, I had a great deal of swelling in my feet. At night, I wore heavy compression stockings and slept with my feet raised on two pillows. Once I began doing this, I found that I urinated more often, which eliminated some of the excess fluid.

IMPORTANT THINGS TO KNOW

In addition to all the ways you can prepare for your baby physically, both your mental approach to childbirth and your support team during this event can help make your birthing experience the best possible one. But don't forget: After the big event, there's a baby to take care of! The end of this section discusses choosing the right professional to check your newborn.

How Preconceptions Affect the Experience of Childbirth

Although women throughout the world give birth through a process of uterine contractions and pushing, we don't all perceive the experience in the same way. How our particular culture frames the idea of birth has as much effect as basic biology does in determining what we will do, think, and feel during and after birth. The environment in which we live, our health-care system, our families and friends, and the support available to us during childbirth will all influence our experiences.

In less westernized parts of the world, women tend to think of birth as a type of work that involves some pain. A laboring woman stays at home, with everyday activities going on around her. She is usually surrounded by female helpers, who physically and emotionally support her during contractions, sometimes share their own birth stories between contractions, and always reinforce the idea that what she is experiencing is normal. When a woman's pain and weariness increase, she is reminded frequently that the baby will soon be born. Birthing pains are not mysterious or frightening, and no one is worried about the mother's ability to withstand her contractions.

Name That Baby (Or Those Babies)

In the United States, today's children have names more diversified than those of earlier generations of children (name conformity peaked around the middle of the last century). The only conformity today seems to be in that most parents want to give their babies unusual names. Whether you're looking for a traditional name or a novel one for your baby, there are a lot of good naming books to help you.

Naming twins may take even more thought than naming a single baby. Twins seem to have less trouble with names when they are not "cutesy" or too much alike. Choose twin names that are equally strong and that sound good together. For fun, here are the top five names of twins in 2016, according to the Social Security Administration.

GIRL/BOY	GIRL/GIRL	BOY/BOY
Madison and Mason	Isabella and Sophia	Jacob and Joshua
Taylor and Tyler	Faith and Hope	Ethan and Evan
Addison and Aiden	Olivia and Sophia	Jayden and Jordan
Emily and Ethan	Ella and Emma	Daniel and David
Emma and Evan	Hailey and Hannah	Ethan and Evan

Western countries have varying approaches to dealing with child-birth pain. Although Denmark and Sweden are literally next door to each other, in the 1980s their attitudes toward birth were quite different. In Denmark, birth was considered a natural process that did not need much interference beyond controlled breathing and massage. On the other hand, the Swedes believed that birth should be entirely painless, with as much pharmacological help as needed to make it so. Women in each country had expectations of their births' being managed in a particular way. When things went as expected, researchers found, both Danish and Swedish women found the experience of childbirth to be positive.

Here in the United States, we have widely divergent approaches to birthing. Childbirth books, classes, and even medical approaches evolve from vastly different viewpoints, many of which directly conflict with one another. The media, health-care practitioners, and child-birth educators often fail to instill in women reasonable expectations of childbirth. What is a woman to think? She may grasp on to a particular viewpoint and conclude that there is one good way to have a baby and that the other approaches are wrong. If her labor then doesn't go as she expected, she may be disappointed with the experience.

It can take some time to figure out what approach to labor is right for you. For some women, reaching deep within themselves to work with and through the pain of labor is of primary importance. For others, being pain-free in labor allows them to let go of their fears and enjoy giving birth. Either natural or medicated birth can be achieved among caring, compassionate people who support the laboring woman.

If you are giving birth in the United States, you have many choices. You can deliver your baby in a hospital, in a birth center, or at home; with medication or without; and generally with whomever you would like to have with you. To be satisfied with the experience, you must be honest with yourself about what is important to you, select a practitioner with whom you feel confident, and make sure you have strong supporters with you during labor. Then you will be able to trust that you will be cared for, make the choices that feel right to you, and feel happy with the baby, the birth, and yourself. As Doña Juana, a Mayan midwife, said in Brigitte Jordan's *Birth in Four Cultures,* every woman must *buscar la forma*—"find her own style."

Letting Labor Unfold

Realistic expectations of birth are general, not specific. You cannot truly know how you will handle an experience you have not yet had, and this is especially true of labor. At the beginning of this chapter, I advised letting go of the desire for complete control. Doing so can make a big difference in your experience of labor. It is good to think through your needs and wishes, but on the day of labor, you must be willing to let the process unfold as it will. This brings me to a subject you may have heard or read about: writing a *birth plan.*

A birth plan is a written description of how a woman wishes, or doesn't wish, her labor to be managed. Years ago, when birth in a hospital was less "family centered," there was a real need for birth plans. Because pregnant women had little open communication with their doctors and nurses, many women made specific written requests to avoid certain hospital procedures that they considered unnecessary.

Today a pregnant or laboring woman has more opportunity to discuss whatever is important to her with the professionals who assist her. She can decide whether she would like to labor with or without pain medications. During labor, as long as she and her baby are fine, she can choose the positions, movements, and coping measures that she finds helpful. She is a full participant in the decision-making process.

In most hospitals today, very few medical procedures are routinely performed on laboring women. The baby's heart rate is monitored at various intervals, but the mother is usually not required to stay in bed during fetal monitoring (page 302); she can sit in a chair and change positions at will. Many hospitals and birth centers now use telemetry monitors (page 302), which make it possible for a mother to walk or even take a shower while her baby's heart rate is being monitored.

Interventions such as the insertion of an intravenous (IV) line, administration of IV fluids, internal fetal monitoring (page 302), and supplementary oxytocin (page 311) are used when the practitioner believes they are necessary for the well-being of mother, baby, or both. For example, if you are vomiting a great deal, you are probably becoming dehydrated. The uterus does not contract effectively if the body is dehydrated. Consequently, IV fluids will make you feel better and will help your contractions be more productive (your nurse can hang your IV on a wheeled stand to allow you to move about freely and even take a shower or bath).

You may sometimes need to listen closely to your doctor, midwife, or nurse to understand why he or she is suggesting a particular action. Ask questions—repeatedly, if necessarily—but realize that safety issues are nonnegotiable. You have selected your doctor or midwife because you believe that he or she is competent to manage the health and safety of you and your baby. Once you are in labor, you must trust this person to take care of you.

Most things typically written in a birth plan can and should be discussed with the practitioner during pregnancy. If you have strong feelings about something having to do with labor, share them with your midwife or doctor. Such a conversation can make a world of difference. I have often heard women say, "I was so worried about _____, but when I spoke with my doctor about it, she explained it so well that she laid my concerns to rest."

Each labor is unique, unpredictable, and outside a woman's conscious control. You will have plenty of work to do in birthing your baby without trying to follow a rigid plan. So let go of any desire to run the show. Trust your body, your partner and other supporters, and your care providers. When you throw out the script, you are likely to have a much more positive birth experience.

Things You May Wish to Discuss with Your Practitioner

As you go through your childbirth course and prepare to give birth, you may have many questions about what to expect from your labor and birth experience. If you have not yet asked your practitioner these questions, now is the time to do so. Write them down before your appointment so that you don't forget them. Here are some things you might want to talk over:

- Will your practitioner definitely attend your delivery? If not, who might take his or her place? Will you be able to meet the substitute practitioner before you give birth?

- At what point in labor should you call your practitioner? When should you go to the hospital or birth center?

- If your water bag breaks or if you go past your due date, how long will your practitioner wait before inducing your labor?

- If your labor must be induced, what method will be used? (See pages 308 to 312.)

- Will you have continuous fetal monitoring, or can it be intermittent? Does your hospital or birth center offer telemetry monitoring or use a hand-held device?

- Will you be automatically subjected to any medical procedures, such intravenous (IV) fluids, the insertion of an IV injection port (in case IV fluids are needed later), or an episiotomy? Or will these be done only if necessary?

- Who can be with you during your labor and birth?

- Will you be able to walk around, change positions, and labor in a shower, regular bath, or whirlpool bath?

- Will you be able to eat and drink in labor?

- What are your practitioner's views on pain medications and anesthesia in labor? Are there any rules regarding how far along you need to be in your labor before using them? Do others in the practice have different rules?

- What are your practitioner's criteria in deciding that a cesarean birth is necessary?

- If you need to have a cesarean, can you elect to be awake and have your partner or other support person with you?

- After the birth, does the baby stay with you or go to the nursery? Can you choose? If the baby does go to the nursery, how long will she need to stay there?

- Can you choose to keep your baby with you continuously after birth, even at night?

- Can your partner stay overnight with you after the baby is born? What sleeping accommodations will be provided for your partner?

- If you are breastfeeding, can you request that your baby not receive any sugar water or formula?

- Will someone help you get started with breastfeeding? Is there a lactation consultant on staff?

- How long can you expect to remain in the hospital or birth center after a vaginal birth? A cesarean birth? Can you go home early, if you choose?

- If you choose to have your baby boy circumcised, when will the procedure be done? Will a topical anesthetic be used? Can you be present?

Choosing Your Baby's Caregiver

The caregiver who will provide health care for your child will become an important person to you and your family. Now is the time to select that person, so you'll be ready to arrange the first checkup soon after the birth.

If you, your partner, or both of you have a family physician—a doctor who provides general health care to both adults and children—she or he can provide your baby's care. If not, you'll want to find out about appropriate practitioners who may be available. You might start by asking for recommendations from your friends, family members, or your obstetrician or midwife.

Your child's health-care provider could be a family physician, a pediatrician (a doctor specializing in the care of children), or a pediatric nurse-practitioner. This specialized nurse-practitioner is a registered nurse who has an advanced degree in the care of children and who practices with a physician.

Many baby doctors no longer grant in-person interviews with expectant parents, but all are happy to answer questions by phone. You will want to make sure that your insurance will cover the practitioner's services. Another important consideration is when he or she will first see your baby. You may also want to ask other questions:

Philosophy of care. What is the caregiver's attitude about preventive care? About alternative medicine such as homeopathy or acupuncture?

Views on infant nutrition. Does the caregiver support breastfeeding? Is there a lactation specialist on staff?

Professional qualifications. Is the caregiver certified by a board in his or her medical specialty?

Accessibility. How easy or difficult is it to reach the caregiver by phone? How far in advance must appointments be scheduled? Where is the office, and how easily can you reach it?

Staff. Are the office staff and nurses friendly and helpful?

Hospital privileges. What hospital would you take the baby to?

Ask Tori, R.N.

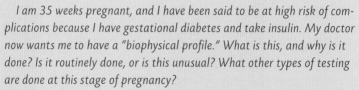

TESTS OF FETAL WELL-BEING

Hi, Tori,

I am 35 weeks pregnant, and I have been said to be at high risk of complications because I have gestational diabetes and take insulin. My doctor now wants me to have a "biophysical profile." What is this, and why is it done? Is it routinely done, or is this unusual? What other types of testing are done at this stage of pregnancy?

—Lilia, Maryland

Dear Lilia,

Fetal testing such as a biophysical profile at this stage is not routine. It is done for a specific reason, such as to check the well-being of an overdue baby (at 41 weeks or beyond) or to assess the functionality of the placenta. Because you have gestational diabetes (page 193), your doctor wants to watch the baby extra closely during these last weeks of your pregnancy.

Three types of fetal tests may be performed at this stage of pregnancy. The first, a *non-stress test*, uses an external electronic fetal monitor to measure the baby's heart rate in response to his own movements. When the baby moves, his heart rate should accelerate by 15 beats per minute for 15 seconds or more. This normally happens at least twice within 20 minutes. If the baby's heartbeat doesn't speed up as expected, a biophysical profile is performed.

A *biophysical profile,* the second type of fetal test, uses ultrasound and has five parts:

- A non-stress test (a second one, if a first has already been performed)
- Measurement of the amount of amniotic fluid around the baby's body
- Observation of the baby's muscle tone (seeing the baby extend an arm or leg and then bring the limb back in toward the body)
- Observation of the baby's large-muscle movements (rolls)

- Observation of the baby's breathing movements (although the baby is not actually breathing, small amounts of fluid move in and out of the lungs with these movements)

This test takes from 20 to 60 minutes to complete. The baby is scored between zero and two points for each part. A total score below eight indicates a need for further testing.

The least common of the three tests, a *Doppler flow study,* uses ultrasound to assess the rate of blood flow in the umbilical blood vein and in the baby's arteries, brain, and heart. The procedure is much like a regular ultrasound exam, except that the test uses color to differentiate the blood vessels. Waveforms on an ultrasound screen show variations in the rate of the blood flow. Decreased flow may indicate that the baby is not receiving enough blood, nutrients, and oxygen from the placenta.

PUPPP (WHAT THE HECK IS IT?)

Tori,

Help! This is my first pregnancy, and I have been miserable for the last several days with a terrible rash and itching. My doctor has diagnosed me with a skin condition called PUPPP. What is this, and is it dangerous?

—April, Michigan

Dear April,

PUPPP stands for *pruritic urticarial papules and plaques of pregnancy* (say that ten times quickly!). Among the many skin rashes that can develop during pregnancy, this one most commonly occurs in abdominal stretch marks but can also occur on the buttocks, thighs, and arms. As you know, PUPPP is itchy, itchy, and itchier. Its cause is unknown, but PUPPP is not a serious condition; it poses no danger to you or your baby. It lasts about six weeks, on average, and disappears within two weeks after birth. It generally doesn't recur, even in subsequent pregnancies.

To lessen the itching, you can try taking oatmeal baths or use an over-the-counter anti-itch cream containing 1 percent hydrocortisone. If this doesn't help, your doctor or midwife may suggest an antihistamine or, if the itching is very severe, a corticosteroid.

BREECH POSITIONS

Dear Tori,

What is the difference between a double footling breech and a complete breech? Our Nicholas has been described as being in both positions.

—Julie, Wyoming

Julie,

A breech baby is positioned buttocks-down rather than head-down in the uterus. The type of breech depends on where the baby's legs are. Let me explain the variations:

Complete breech. The baby is in a sitting position, with his legs crossed.

Frank breech. The baby's legs are straight up, folded flat against his face. His arms may be around the legs.

Footling breech. One leg is fully extended; the other is folded under.

Double footling breech. Both legs are fully extended. Another unusual position is *transverse.* In this case, the baby lies horizontally, across the uterus.

Babies move around a great deal in the uterus and are likely to be in many positions over the course of a pregnancy. Your baby could have been in a complete breech position at one time and could have extended a leg into a footling position at another time.

During the last few weeks of pregnancy, a baby usually settles down into one position. This is most likely to be vertex, or head-down, although some babies do settle into a breech or transverse position. Any of these non-head-down positions makes vaginal delivery more dangerous. If your baby is breech at 37 weeks and you want to avoid a cesarean, external version (page 230) is definitely worth a try.

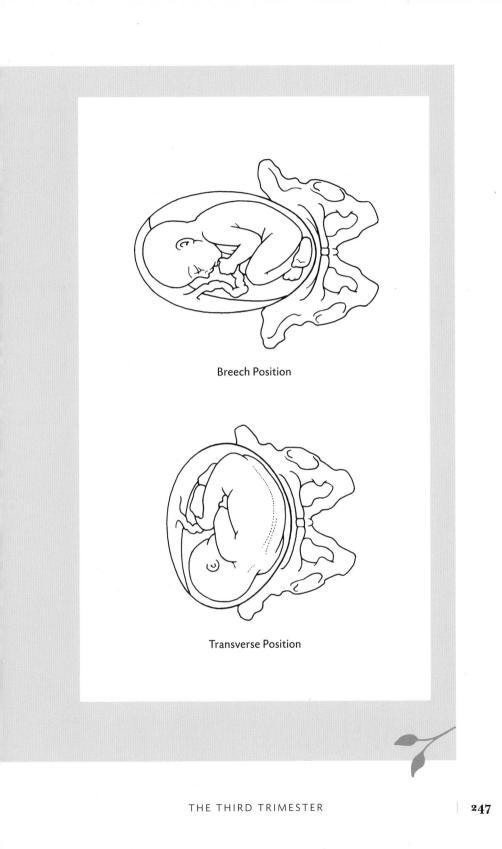

Breech Position

Transverse Position

MORNING SICKNESS IN THE EIGHTH MONTH?

Tori,

I am just now 32 weeks, and I have suddenly developed awful heartburn and really awful episodes of upset stomach. I wake up in the middle of the night with the urge to vomit. Is this normal? I never had any morning sickness. Could I have developed it this late in my pregnancy?

—Vanessa, Mississippi

Vanessa,

As your baby and your uterus grow, the pressure upward on your stomach increases. This causes stomach acids to back up into your esophagus. The condition may also cause sudden vomiting, without the lingering nausea that is usual with morning sickness.

Here are some tips that other women have found helpful for heartburn and vomiting in late pregnancy:

- Eat smaller, more frequent meals.
- Avoid spicy, acidic, or fatty foods.
- Don't eat immediately before bedtime; stay upright for a time after each meal.
- Take a walk after meals to promote digestion.
- Take Tums or another antacid.

Be sure you let your practitioner know about this problem. He or she may recommend an antacid and offer some additional suggestions for relief.

SPONTANEOUS RUPTURE OF THE WATER BAG

Hi, Tori!

I've heard that only a small percentage of women actually have their "bag of waters" break prior to labor. With my first child, my amniotic sac ruptured at 29 weeks and I delivered at 31 weeks. There was no known cause, such as infection, for the premature rupture. Now I am 32 weeks along in my second pregnancy, and preterm labor began in my 26th week. I am doing very well, taking terbutaline tablets, and staying on bed rest. Could my water bag break before this baby's birth, too?

—Rebecca, North Carolina

Rebecca,

Your question concerns two topics: the rupture of the water bag (amniotic sac) before labor begins, and premature labor. Let's address these two separately.

In the movies, labor always seems to begin with the breaking of the water bag. But labor actually begins this way for only 10 to 15 percent of women. When it does, it usually happens at full term, between 37 and 41 weeks.

Labor seldom begins before 37 weeks. But when it does, it often begins with rupture of the membranes. Sometimes, there has been a mild infection in the uterus and amniotic sac. This condition, called *chorioamnionitis,* can be difficult to diagnose and treat. In other cases, undiagnosed cervical dilation has caused the amniotic sac to break. In still others, the amniotic membrane was weak for some reason.

The fact that your water bag ruptured prematurely in your first pregnancy does not necessarily mean it will this time. Although both the premature birth of your first baby and the premature labor you have experienced in this pregnancy increase the likelihood that you'll deliver prematurely again, the terbutaline and bed rest appear to be working well for you. Hang in there for just a few more weeks!

WHAT IS A DOULA?

Hi, Tori,

My wife has said that she wants to check into the possibility of having a doula with us at our baby's birth. I am not familiar with the use of doulas, and I would like to know more about them. I am afraid that I won't be as involved if we have one. What are your thoughts?

—David, Arkansas

Dear David,

Many women wish to have only their partner, practitioner, and nurse present at their baby's birth. Others want extra support, perhaps because of a previous difficult labor or general anxiety about giving birth. Some couples ask a close friend or a family member to accompany them. Others hire a trained labor assistant, or doula (from a Greek word for "woman's helper"). A doula provides continuous physical, emotional, and informational support to mothers and their partners during labor and birth. Studies have shown that continuous labor support decreases the use of pain medication, epidural anesthesia, episiotomies, and cesarean sections and provides greater feelings of control and satisfaction for women in labor.

A doula would play a unique role on your birth team. She would not replace your own loving support for your partner. Instead, she could help both of you by offering suggestions about comfort measures—such as relaxation, visualization, breathing, massage, aromatherapy, use of a birthing ball, and spending time in the tub or shower—and assistance in carrying out these measures. She would not influence any medical decisions that you and your partner may need to make, but she could help you figure out what questions to ask of your practitioner and your nurse to help you in making these decisions. Each person on the birth team has different responsibilities, and everyone working together makes the amazing dance of labor a very positive experience for the mother and her partner.

Your doctor, midwife, childbirth educator, or hospital or birth center staff may be able to help you find a doula. These are some good questions to ask the person you're considering hiring:

- What sort of training and experience do you have?
- What is your personal philosophy about childbirth and labor support?
- What are your feelings about the use of anesthesia and other medications in labor?
- What practitioners have you worked with, and are you familiar with ours?
- Are you familiar with our hospital or birth center? Can you share with us any experiences that you have had with the facility?
- When do you typically arrive during your client's labor? Do you come to our home or meet us at the hospital or birth center?
- Do you work with other doulas who serve as substitutes when you are not available?
- What is your fee? Do we need to make a partial payment before the birth? Will you refund our money if you are unable to attend the birth?
- When can we meet, so that we can get to know you and you can get to know us?

You might also ask the doula to provide references.

The cost of using a doula can vary a great deal. The community hospital in my neighborhood provides free doula services to women who have no partner, friend, or relative to accompany them in labor. Doulas usually charge for their work, however, and depending on where you live, I have seen fees ranging from $350 to more than $2,000.

Starting Labor with a Splash

For 15 years, I had told my PillowTalk moms that the chance of a water bag's breaking in public was truly next to nothing. Then, five days before Alexander was due, I was shopping for Christmas lights in a black, billowy maternity dress. As I was standing in the store aisle, I felt a little pinch, and suddenly on the floor was one of the biggest puddles of amniotic fluid I had ever seen. I stood there for a second, stunned, and then ran out of the store, laughing hysterically and dripping all the way out the front door. I was glad I was wearing a dress with so much fabric, which soaked up some of the water. Then the contractions started, and within a couple of hours, I was in booming labor. What I'd always said rarely happened had happened to me!

DAD'S CORNER

For months now, your partner's belly has been preceding her into the room and perhaps nudging you out of bed. Your mate may be experiencing sleep disturbances, fatigue, or feelings of worry and wonder—and you may be as well. For you, labor and birth may seem too big to be real, or too real to escape. One new dad expressed the feeling well: "While hugging my wife, I looked down at her enormous belly, and I suddenly realized that this was going to happen—no matter what." Congratulations! You are having your own labor pains, which push thoughts and feelings of parenthood into the forefront of your mind. And they are right on time. During this second-to-last month, the amazement and anxiety associated with pregnancy naturally become more intense. While a mom may worry about what her labor is going to be like, a dad may worry about the health of his mate and baby.

With all the focus on the mom and baby, some men feel like a fifth wheel at this point. You might think you can have no effect on what your partner will experience. Don't believe it! The bond and harmony between parents greatly affects the mother's attitude toward birth, breastfeeding, and the baby. Studies have shown that the more involved Dad is, the higher satisfaction Mom reports in moving from pregnancy to birth to parenting. You can help ease your partner's way by participating in prenatal classes, visiting the doctor or midwife with her, and helping her with preparations for the baby.

You may be worrying about how you'll respond to your partner's labor. It can be very hard to watch a loved one suffer discomfort, fear, or pain. For most of us, feeling we have no control over a situation increases our anxiety. But you won't have to feel helpless during labor. In the next chapter, I'll describe specific ways you can support your partner. For now, know that your presence, your love, and your attention to her experience have a huge effect on her sense of security.

Appreciate, too, your direct importance to your baby. You are one of the two people who will serve as your child's main models in life. Value what you have to offer.

Treat Her Well. Take your partner swimming; water can really take the weight off her feet. Be sure to choose a place where she is comfortable—perhaps a friend's private pool or a community pool when few people are around.

Tori's Tip: Relax!

Relaxation is the key to coping with contractions. Relaxing in spite of pain is a skill that can be learned, and it can be applied not only during labor but also in any other stressful situation. No matter how busy your life is, if you can commit to a brief practice time each day, you will add an invaluable skill to your labor tool-kit.

You may not know how it feels to be fully relaxed. Doing the following exercise once or twice daily can teach you to distinguish tension from relaxation. It is important to feel your muscles relax and soften rather than to just think about this.

Put on some soft, recorded music, and then find a comfortable position that will allow all your muscles to relax completely. You might lie in a semi-reclining position with pillows under your knees and arms. Or you might lie on your side with a pillow between your knees, one in front of you with your arm draped over it, and another pillow supporting your head.

Close your eyes, and think of a place or color that is restful to you. Or, locate a focal point two to four feet from your eyes. Breathe slowly and deeply, in through your nose (unless it is stuffy) and out through your mouth.

Taking one area at a time, from toes to head, contract the muscles of your body for a count of two, and then slowly let the muscles go limp and loose, paying attention to the feeling of releasing tension. Here is a sequence you can follow.

1. Pull your toes down, and then relax.
2. Pull your toes up, and then relax.
3. Turn your ankles out, and then relax.
4. Bend your knees slightly, and then relax.
5. Extend your left leg out, and then relax.
6. Extend your right leg out, and then relax.
7. Tighten your buttocks, and then relax.
8. Tighten your pelvic-floor muscles (do a Kegel), and then relax.
9. Expand your abdominal muscles, and then relax.
10. Make fists, and then relax.
11. Extend your fingers, and then relax.

12. Bend your wrists down, and then relax.
13. Bend your wrists up, and then relax.
14. Straighten your elbows, and then relax.
15. Raise your shoulders, and then relax.
16. Squeeze your chest muscles, and then relax.
17. Expand your chest, and then relax.
18. Pull your shoulder blades forward, and then relax.
19. Pull your shoulder blades back, and then relax.
20. Arch your lower back, and then relax.
21. Bend your neck forward, and then relax.
22. Tighten your jaw, and then relax.
23. Raise your eyebrows, and then relax.
24. Squeeze your facial muscles, and then relax.

Now take another deep, slow breath, and slowly exhale. Lie still for a few more moments to be mindful of the wonder of your child and to enjoy the sensation of full relaxation. Be aware of what it feels like to be limp, loose, and heavy. Just as tension can spread throughout your body, so can relaxation

All about Labor

YOUR NINTH MONTH: WEEKS 36 THROUGH 40 (OR 41 AND COUNTING...)

IN THIS VERY EXUBERANT, ANXIOUS MONTH, everything is gearing toward the birth of your child. The anticipation is exhilarating and tiring. Waiting is not easy, and especially if your pregnancy goes past your due date, the last few days or weeks can go by slowly. Enjoy them! This is your last opportunity to get everything ready and to spend quiet time with your mate. Treasure the days until you two become three (or more).

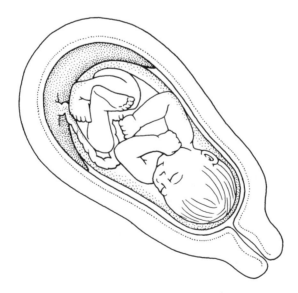

WHAT'S HAPPENING WITH YOUR BABY?

I hear the same question from a lot of moms around this time in their pregnancies: "How can my belly possibly get any bigger?" You may be surprised by how much your belly will change over these next few weeks. During this month, the baby will gain about ½ pound (226 g) a week. She may gain 2 more pounds (900 g) between the start of this month and the day she is born!

These last few weeks are important for your baby in another way. At the beginning of this month, she is developing in her lungs a substance called *surfactant*, which is necessary for her to breathe properly and for her lungs to stay inflated. Once surfactant has developed, she is ready for the outside world. At 37 weeks, her lungs will be mature and ready to function on their own, she will be considered full-term, and you will be able to safely deliver at any time.

Also in the last month, the baby may "drop" lower in the abdomen or pelvis in a head-down position. You may have heard this referred to as *lightening*. It can happen two weeks before you go into labor or after your labor begins.

Your baby may be covered with *vernix*, a thick, creamy coating that protects baby's skin in your amnotic fluid, and *lanugo*, soft, downy hair. The soles of the feet have creases, and if the baby is a boy, the testes will fully descend into his scrotal sac this month.

WHAT'S HAPPENING WITH YOUR BODY?

New things keep happening. Your belly button may now stick out. As the baby is taking up nearly all the room in your abdomen, your other organs are feeling the squeeze. You may feel short of breath or sore under your ribs. You probably have to pee more often because the baby is pressing on your bladder. If you have had heartburn, it may be more noticeable now, and you may not be able to eat a full meal at one time. You may also notice more swelling in your ankles, feet, and hands.

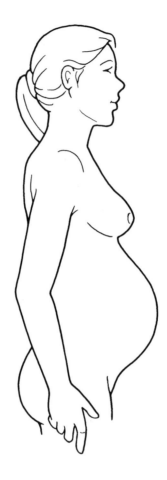

Shortness of Breath

If you're like many women in late pregnancy, you may be feeling as though you can't get enough air. What causes this feeling? Your diaphragm—the broad, flat muscle that lies under your lungs—is being pushed upward by your expanding uterus. The diaphragm rises about 1½ inches (4 cm) from its usual position during late pregnancy. This may seem like a small amount, but it's enough to decrease your lung capacity.

At the same time, the hormone progesterone is acting on the respiratory center in the brain, causing you to breathe more deeply. As a result, although your total lung capacity is decreased, you are actually taking in more air with each breath than you normally did before your pregnancy.

Despite the discomfort you may feel, you don't need to worry about your baby. Your expanded respiratory and circulatory systems are seeing to it that the baby is getting plenty of oxygen. Your body is now carrying more blood and more oxygen-rich hemoglobin. These increases cause the oxygen level in your blood to go up, ensuring an adequate supply to your growing baby.

Keeping your back as straight as possible will help your breathing. Practice sitting or standing with your back straight and your shoulders back, relaxed, and down. When sleeping, lie propped up on pillows or on your side to lessen the pressure on your diaphragm. If none of these measures help, hang in there. Your breathing may improve if your baby drops farther down in your pelvis before labor, but if this doesn't happen, know that like many other pregnancy discomforts, this one will go away immediately or quite shortly after birth.

If your breathing problems are severe, check with your practitioner. They could be a sign of a more serious problem such as asthma.

Your Prenatal Checkups

You'll now be seeing your doctor or midwife once a week. Your blood pressure and weight will be checked, as will the baby's movements. Your practitioner will continue to measure the length of your uterus (from your pubic bone to your fundus) and listen to your baby's heart. In addition, as your due date draws near, the practitioner will determine the position of the baby.

Approximately 97 percent of babies settle into a vertex (head-down) position by the ninth month. Your doctor can feel the position of your baby's body with a series of hand movements (called Leopold's Maneuvers) on your abdomen. He or she may also be able to feel the baby's head (or another "presenting" part, if the baby is not head-down) during a vaginal exam.

At about the 36th week, your practitioner will swab your vagina and anus and then have the specimen tested for group B streptococcus (or group B strep, or GBS). About 25 percent of women test positive for GBS. Testing positive does not mean that you have an infection; the bacteria live in the vagina and rectum and cause no harm to you. But if you were to get a uterine infection with GBS, your baby could also become infected. A GBS infection in a newborn is very serious. Although such infections are uncommon, it is recommended that all pregnant women who test positive for GBS be given intravenous antibiotics during active labor, usually every four hours. This preventive measure has dramatically decreased the number of babies affected by the illness.

At about the 39th week, many health-care providers perform a vaginal exam. Three conditions of your pregnancy are assessed at this time, as described in the following sections.

CERVICAL EFFACEMENT

The cervix, or the opening to the uterus, is situated at the top of the vagina. In many women, the cervix is easy to feel with the fingers, but in other women, it is quite high in the vagina and behind the top of the baby's head. In this arrangement, called a *posterior* cervix, the cervix is more difficult to reach. The cervix usually feels a lot like the soft side of your thumb, from the tip to your first knuckle. Before labor with a first baby, the cervix is generally between 2 and 5 centimeters long and quite firm. In a subsequent pregnancy, it can be much shorter and softer.

Effacement is the thinning of the cervix. As it effaces, the cervix softens and shortens. A "ripe" cervix is soft and beginning to thin. Your practitioner will refer to the effacement of your cervix in terms of a percentage. For example, if your cervix is 30 percent effaced, it is about one-third shorter than before pregnancy. The cervix must be 100 percent effaced, or paper-thin, before it begins to *dilate*, or open.

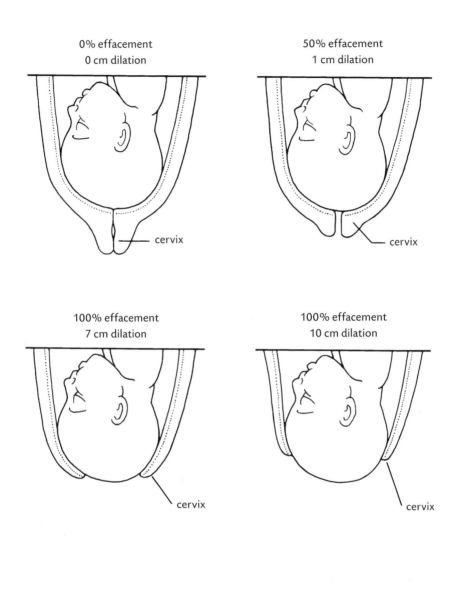

0% effacement
0 cm dilation

cervix

50% effacement
1 cm dilation

cervix

100% effacement
7 cm dilation

cervix

100% effacement
10 cm dilation

cervix

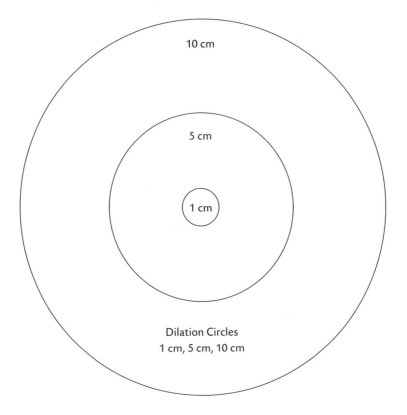

10 cm

5 cm

1 cm

Dilation Circles
1 cm, 5 cm, 10 cm

CERVICAL DILATION

The cervix seldom dilates much before labor begins, especially with a first baby. Still, any dilation after 37 weeks is considered normal.

Dilation is measured in centimeters, from 0 centimeters, or closed, to 10. At 10 centimeters, the cervix is completely dilated and has moved around the baby's head. (Ten centimeters is an approximate measurement; babies' heads do vary in size.) Once the cervix is completely dilated, the pushing phase of labor begins.

STATION

This term refers to the location of the baby's presenting part, usually the head, in relation to the pelvis. (If the baby is breech at 37 weeks, a doctor will probably perform an external version, as described on page 230.)

When the baby's forehead is even with the inner, bony prominences

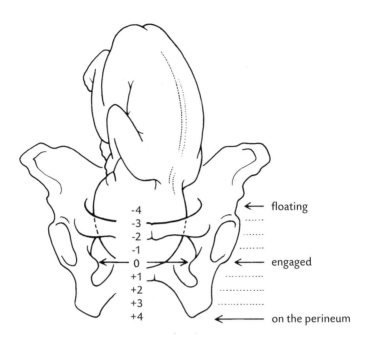

-4
-3
-2
-1
0 ← engaged
+1
+2
+3
+4

← floating

← on the perineum

of the pelvic bones (*ischial spines*), the baby is "engaged" in the pelvis at 0 station. Other stations are numbered in centimeters above or below 0 station. For example, if the baby is 1 centimeter above the ischial spines, he is at -1 station. Most women, especially first-time moms, go into labor with the baby between 0 and -2 station.

How Can You Know When Labor Will Start?

Until your labor actually begins, no measurement of effacement, station, or dilation can tell you how soon it will happen. A woman who is 3 centimeters dilated for weeks may not deliver until after her due date, and another woman, this one with a long, closed cervix, may go into labor the next day. For many women who have just been told that they won't go into labor for weeks, labor then begins—contrarily, it seems—the next day. My own labor started suddenly. The day before Alexander was born, my cervix was completely firm, long, and closed, and my doctor remarked that my body wasn't in too much of a hurry. Sixteen hours later, my waters broke and I was in labor. Within a couple of hours after that, my cervix was completely effaced and 4 centimeters dilated. You just never know.

Although it is a continuous process, labor is generally discussed in terms of stages. There are four of these, the last being the immediate postpartum period, after the baby is born. Although nothing in labor is the same for everyone, the stages of labor, especially for a first-time mom, are fairly clear-cut. Knowing where you are in each stage is a little more complicated.

Labor: An Overview

For 75 percent of women giving birth for the first time, labor lasts between 14 and 24 hours (subsequent labors tend to be significantly shorter). Now, before you get nervous about this, let's see how that time breaks down into stages and phases. Keep in mind that the times shown here apply to most women, but not all. One in four will have a shorter or longer labor.

1. *First stage: effacement and dilation*, 13 to 21 hours. The cervix fully effaces and dilates to 10 centimeters, over the course of several phases:

• *Early or latent phase*, 8 to 12 hours. The cervix reaches full effacement and 3 centimeters' dilation.

• *Active phase*, 4 to 6 hours. The cervix reaches from 3 to 7 centimeters' dilation.

• *Transition phase*, 1 to 3 hours. It widens further, from 7 to 10 centimeters' dilation.

2. *Second stage: pushing*, 1 to 3 hours. The baby is pushed through the birth canal. This stage ends in birth. Larger babies generally take longer to push out than small babies.

3. *Third stage: birth of the placenta*, 5 to 20 minutes. This is generally not difficult and is minimally uncomfortable.

4. *Fourth stage: immediate postpartum*, 2 hours. During this time, the mom is carefully observed to be sure her uterus is contracting, her bleeding is under control, and she is getting attached to her baby. This is a time for her to rest, eat and drink as she wishes, and breastfeed her baby.

The following pages describe the stages of labor in more detail.

First Stage: Effacement and Dilation

In this stage of labor, your cervix begins to change in shape. Irregular contractions of the uterus are pulling the cervix toward the baby's head. The contractions and the pressure from the baby begin to flatten, or thin, the cervix.

EARLY OR LATENT PHASE

Some labors begin fast and furiously, essentially skipping this phase. In others, this phase may pass unnoticed. But most women, especially first-time moms, experience a long warm-up period in the beginning of labor. Knowing that there might be a long latent phase can help you pace yourself physically, mentally, and emotionally. In classes, I try to help women think about this 8- to 12-hour phase as the body's preparation for the tough work of active labor ahead.

You may be in early labor for several hours before you realize that labor has begun. Here are some signs that labor is starting:

- *Nagging backache, or achiness in the lower abdomen or legs.*
- *Menstrual-like cramps.*
- *Loose bowels.*
- *A vague feeling that you are "coming down with something" or ate something that didn't agree with you.* I can't tell you how many women have told me that they thought they were getting the stomach flu when they were going into labor.
- *A mucous or bloody vaginal discharge.* The "mucous plug," the thick mucus contained in the cervix during pregnancy, may loosen and come out when the cervix begins thinning and opening. When tinged with blood, the mucous plug is called a "bloody show." You may notice this reddish brown discharge when you wipe yourself after using the toilet. The slight bleeding is caused by the breakage of the small capillaries of the cervix. (If you ever notice bright red bleeding, call your practitioner, as it could be coming from your placenta.)
- *Rupture of the membranes (amniotic sac).* This can happen with either a large gush of fluid—a cup or more—or a constant trickle. In either case, let your doctor or midwife know. Breaking your bag of waters doesn't necessarily mean you will go immediately into labor. About 50 percent of women whose membranes rupture before labor go into labor within 12 hours; the other 50 percent do not.

Once the membranes rupture, there is some risk that bacteria could travel up into your uterus and cause an infection. This risk increases sharply after 24 hours. If you don't go into labor within a certain number of hours, usually no more than 24, your doctor or midwife will recommend that your labor be induced (ask your practitioner what his or her policy is). If you have tested positive for group B strep, your labor will be induced as soon as it is clear that your amniotic sac has broken.

Your doctor or midwife will want to know what color the leaking fluid is. It should be clear or slightly pink. If it has any yellow or green coloring, then it contains meconium, the baby's stool (page 158). A baby who passes meconium before birth may be postterm (past 40 weeks' gestation) or experiencing some stress in the uterus. The main concern with meconium in the amniotic fluid, though, is that if the baby were to inhale some of the meconium-tinged fluid at birth, he could develop a serious respiratory illness. For this reason, the mother's practitioner or a pediatrician gently suctions the baby's mouth and nose at birth.

Extra energy. Some women experience a "nesting urge," or a burst of energy in the day or so before labor begins. This feeling may give you an indication that things are going to get started soon, but it isn't a reliable sign that labor is actually beginning. If you feel especially perky, try not to clean the garage; you're going to need this energy!

During early labor, your cervix is doing all of its thinning and effacing. Your contractions occur irregularly and vary in strength. During the first several hours, you may notice a low backache or slight crampy feeling that increases over time. This backache or crampiness may come

What Are "Irregularly Regular" Contractions?

What I call irregularly regular contractions happen during early labor and are sometimes uncomfortable, but they're not consistent in their frequency or strength. For example, you might have contractions 6 minutes apart for 30 minutes. Then for the next 30 minutes, they may space out to 12 or 15 minutes apart. Some may be strong; some you may barely notice. They tell you that your engine is warming up.

and go. It may last for a few seconds and then stop. A hallmark of this time is inconsistency; I like to refer to early-labor contractions as "irregularly regular." As the hours pass, the cramps become more pronounced, regular, and frequent.

The best way to get through this time is to play down the fact that your body is going into labor. Remind yourself that this is the warm-up phase. If you can, do whatever is normal for you for the time of day. Distraction and diversions are excellent coping tools for this phase. If you become uncomfortable, just change or stop what you are doing. In the daytime, you might do any of these things:

- Eat lightly.
- Pack your bag for the hospital or birth center.
- Go for a walk. Do a couple of errands, perhaps to arrange for the care of your pets. Being upright and walking helps to keep contractions coming. Don't exhaust yourself, though.
- Go see a movie.

With any of these activities, I suggest including your partner. If he is at work, you might call him as soon as you suspect this is the big day, or you might wait until the signs of labor are more obvious. Couples tell me lovely stories of the things they did together during early labor.

If it is nighttime, try these suggestions:

- Sleep, if possible. You may not be sleeping all that much now, anyway, but any amount of sleep you can catch is good—even catnaps.
- Take a warm bath or shower.
- Read or watch TV. Keep the lights low, so that you may doze some.

Being as well rested as possible will help immensely in labor.

During early labor, you may be quite uncomfortable at times, but you will cope better with the strong contractions of active labor if you don't feel as though you have already been laboring for hours. Put off using your breathing techniques and other labor coping tools and support measures until you really need them. Focusing too much on the mild contractions of early labor can tire you, your partner, and any other support people you have with you.

What to Pack for the Hospital or Birth Center

You won't need much. Today, it is unusual for a woman to spend more than two days in the hospital after a vaginal birth or more than three to four days after a cesarean birth. Most hospitals and birth centers provide basic supplies such as juice, ice, comfortable gowns, towels, washcloths, and materials to make hot or cold packs. Many also send new parents home with items such as sanitary pads, diapers, an infant stocking cap, an infant T-shirt, and a receiving blanket. Check with your hospital or birth center about what will be provided; you might need to bring some of these items from home. In addition, you will want to bring some of these:

FOR MOM

- Bathrobe and slippers
- Basic toiletry items (toothbrush, hairbrush, hair clip or hair band)
- Favorite socks
- Breath spray or breath mints
- Lip balm
- Massage oil
- Massage aid (although your partner's hand will work fine)
- Comfortable pillow (with a case that isn't white, so you don't forget to bring it home)
- Frozen ice or juice bars, or your favorite juice or other cold drink
- Small cooler (if no refrigerator will be available)
- Music player or laptop for music streaming. Check if your birth place has the ability to stream music. If not, you may need to make a playlist.
- Reading material, magazines, laptop, or a deck of cards (especially helpful if you are having your labor induced)
- Nursing bra (if you already have one)
- Extra pair of underpants
- Loose, comfortable clothes for going home (you could wear the same outfit home that you arrive in)

FOR THE PARTNER

- Simple, nourishing snack food
- Basic toiletry items
- Change of clothes (all clothes should be comfortable and easy to move in)
- Swimming suit (in case you want to go into the shower or bath with Mom)
- Phone and battery charger (labeled so that you remember to take it home)
- Video or still camera (if you want to take more detailed photos and videos than with your phone). Hospitals do not allow videos to be taken of medical or surgical procedures, but you can certainly take them of the baby!

FOR THE BABY

- Outfit for the trip home
- Warm blanket (if the weather is cold)
    If you would like to walk home, check with your hospital to see if they have a policy regarding carrying your baby home in an appropriate carrier. If you are driving or taking a ride service home, you'll need to have the base and car seat installed in that vehicle for the trip.

Frequently timing contractions is neither necessary nor helpful. Timing your contractions for hours can make you crazy and does not help to pass the time. There are lots of nifty phone apps available to time contractions. *Do not download them!* How can you distract yourself from your contractions if you are timing them?

The most common reason for contractions that don't increase in strength or frequency is dehydration. Some other signs of dehydration are a dry or sticky mouth, lethargy, lack of stamina, and concentrated, dark yellow urine. If you become better hydrated, prodromal contractions (page 272) may stop completely, or you may move on to active labor. *Staying well hydrated can dramatically decrease the likelihood of prodromal labor.*

As you are nearing active labor, you will eventually want to time a few of your contractions, just to see where you are. At this point, you should time both the length of each contraction, from beginning to end, and the frequency of the contractions—that is, the length of time from the beginning of one contraction to the beginning of the next. For example, if one contraction starts at 8:00 and lasts until 8:01, and the next one begins at 8:05 and lasts until 8:06, the two contractions are 1 minute long each and 5 minutes apart.

Tori's Tip: Put Off Packing Your Bag

Some women pack a bag to take to the hospital or birth center weeks in advance of labor. It's a good idea to think ahead about what you would like to take, but the actual packing is a perfect activity to help keep you occupied during the warm-up phase of labor. It is unlikely that your baby will come so quickly that you won't be able to finish packing, and if this happens, your partner or someone else can always retrieve what you need later. For advice about what to pack, see page 268 to 269.

When you have been having strong contractions coming 5 minutes apart, lasting at least 1 minute each, 1 full hour (the 5-1-1 Recipe), and you are unable to walk, talk, or socialize in any way during the contractions, you are very likely beginning active labor. If you are planning a hospital or birth center birth, this is probably the time to go in (call your doctor or midwife first, though; this could save you an unnecessary trip). You are likely to arrive with your cervix 2 to 3 centimeters dilated, with plenty of time to settle in before your baby is born. Waiting this long won't prevent you from having an epidural or other pain medication, if you choose to.

If your contractions don't yet follow the 5-1-1 Recipe, try to wait another hour or so before going to the hospital. Time your contractions again, if you need to. Actually, when you are unable to walk or talk through contractions that are coming every few minutes, you won't need your wristwatch to know that you are in active labor!

The main purpose of the 5-1-1 Recipe is to help you avoid going to the hospital too early, as many couples do. Time may seem to slow down once you arrive at the hospital or birth center. If you go in before you are in active labor, you will probably be sent home. It can be reassuring to be examined and know that everything is fine, but it can also be disappointing to go to the hospital prepared to have your baby and then come home still pregnant. If you aren't sent home, you will be at greater risk of medical interventions for a prolonged latent phase of labor. Going to the hospital too early can even increase your risk of a cesarean.

Under the following circumstances, you should call your practitioner or go to the hospital (or both) before your contractions follow the 5-1-1 Recipe:

Your first contractions are at least 1 minute long and less than 5 minutes apart. In this case, you may be having a very fast labor. Women who have fast labors tend to skip or not notice early labor.

- Your membranes rupture, and the amniotic fluid is green or dark yellow.
- Your membranes rupture, and you have tested positive for group B strep (page 260).

What Is False Labor?

Uncomfortable contractions occurring over a long period without changing into the stronger and more regular ones of active labor are known as prodromal, or false, labor. These contractions are typically short (less than 30 seconds) in duration, and they don't become stronger over time. They can make you very tired and discouraged.

- You have heavy bleeding or unremitting, severe pain.
- You are extremely uncomfortable, afraid, or worried.

You should also call your practitioner if your membranes rupture but labor pains don't begin right away. Even if you have tested negative for group B strep and the amniotic fluid is clear, you and your doctor or midwife need to discuss strategy. You will probably remain home for a specific time or until you are in labor.

In general, there is no need to call your practitioner under these circumstances:

- You have cramps or irregular contractions, even if some are strong. In this case, you are probably still in early labor.
- You notice a slightly bloody or a mucous discharge and you are not yet having regular contractions.
- You are managing your contractions well at home.

If you live close to your hospital or birth center, you may choose to stay home for a while even if your contractions are 5 minutes or less apart (just be sure to let your practitioner know what is going on). For two women whose labors last the same length of time, the one who spends less time in the hospital or birth center generally reports feeling as though her labor were shorter and describes her overall experience as more positive.

During the latent phase of labor, about 25 percent of women experience back labor. Usually when labor begins, the baby is in the *anterior* position, facing her mother's back. In this position, the baby's head flexes more easily under the pubic bone and through the pelvis. When back labor occurs, however, the baby has settled into the pelvis in the posterior position, facing the same way as her mother. In this position, the hard back of the baby's skull presses directly against the bones of the mother's back. The pressure of bone on bone can be very uncomfortable. You may feel as though all your contractions are in your very low back or between your buttocks. Firm back massage and getting on your hands and knees are most helpful in taking the pressure off your back. Sitting in a bathtub or whirlpool bath or standing in the shower with the full stream of water on the pressure spot can also relieve the pain. About 90 percent of the time, a baby in the posterior position will turn into the optimal anterior position during active labor.

Tori's Tip:
Go to the Hospital Only When
Active Labor Has Begun

How do you know when you are in active labor?
Follow the 5-1-1 Recipe:

Your contractions should come
5 minutes apart.
1 They should last 1 minute each.
1 These have continued for 1 full hour.

The most important piece of the 5-1-1 recipe is that *every* contraction is one that you are *unable* to walk or talk through. This is generally a good recipe for choosing when to head in to the hospital or birth center or when to have the midwife come for a home birth. Your practitioner may give you a different recipe, though, especially if you have already had a baby.

If you live close to your hospital or birth center, you may choose to stay home for a while even if your contractions are 5 minutes or less apart (just be sure to let your practitioner know what is going on). For two women whose labors last the same length of time, the one who spends less time in the hospital or birth center generally reports feeling as though her labor were shorter and describes her overall experience as more positive.

During the latent phase of labor, about 25 percent of women experience back labor. Usually when labor begins, the baby is in the *anterior* position, facing her mother's back. In this position, the baby's head flexes more easily under the pubic bone and through the pelvis. When back labor occurs, however, the baby has settled into the pelvis in the *posterior* position, facing the same way as her mother. In this position, the hard back of the baby's skull presses directly against the bones of the mother's back. The pressure of bone on bone can be very uncomfortable. You may feel as though all your contractions are in your very low back or between your buttocks. Firm back massage and getting on your hands and knees are most helpful in taking the pressure off your back. Sitting in a bathtub or whirlpool bath or standing in the shower with the full stream of water on the pressure spot can also relieve the pain. About 90 percent of the time, a baby in the posterior position will turn into the optimal anterior position during active labor.

ACTIVE PHASE

This phase occurs when the engine has fully kicked into gear. The first sign that you are moving into this stage is that you will probably lose your sense of humor, completely. Believe it or not, this is a pretty accurate way of determining that you are moving into the "working" phase of labor. You may be uncomfortable and somewhat anxious during early labor, but you will be able to distract yourself and perhaps maintain a bit of lightness. You will probably become much quieter and internally focused as you approach active labor.

At this time, your cervix is dilating from 3 to 6 centimeters. Your contractions are regular and increasing in frequency; before long,

What Does a Good, Strong Labor Contraction Feel Like?

A good, strong contraction feels very much like a leg cramp—a charley horse—only it is in the center of your body. Working diligently to dilate your cervix, the uterus gets just as hard as your leg muscle gets when you have a leg cramp. Once you have felt a charley-horse contraction, there is no mistaking that you are in active labor!

they will be 2 to 3 minutes apart. They probably continue to last about 1 minute, and they may take your breath away. Distraction no longer works. A hallmark of active labor is that *every contraction is one that you cannot talk or walk through.* You may need to stop moving, stand against the wall, or sit down during contractions.

It helps to keep in mind (or to be reminded by your partner or someone else) that contractions are not continuous. They do not go on forever. No matter how difficult a contraction may be, it always ends, and then you get a break. Knowing that a contraction will last only 60 to 75 seconds can help you to deal with even the most difficult ones. After each contraction, you can talk, change positions, take a drink, and get ready to deal with the next one.

Your coping measures of relaxation, controlled breathing, and support from your partner can be very helpful now. Here are some specific ways to cope:

Keep your shoulders loose and your body as relaxed as possible. Many women do this naturally when they get into a very focused state. Keeping your body loose and limp helps your uterus to work more efficiently and helps you better manage your contractions.

Fear, Tension, and Pain

Each of these—fear, tension, and pain—increases the likelihood of the others, and sometimes it is hard to know which comes first. We do know that you can break the cycle of fear, tension, and pain in labor. Knowledge, reassurance, relaxation, and support help to decrease all of them.

Try different positions for comfort. See "Positions for Comfort," below.

Focus on your breathing. See "Breathing for Labor," page 281.

Take one contraction at a time.

Drink liquids, suck ice chips, or have a juice bar. It is important that you remain well hydrated during labor.

Take a bath (regular or whirlpool) or a shower. Your practitioner may prefer that you not take a bath if your water bag has broken, but a shower is generally permitted. I have found that many women actually prefer the shower; the water spray on the belly or back can relieve pressure and decrease the intensity of contractions. Water is wonderful for laboring!

Ask for a massage wherever it feels good. For specific ideas, see "Dad's Corner," page 320.

Positions for comfort. In early labor, standing and walking may have helped keep your contractions coming. In active labor, though, your uterus is doing all the work, and you have strong contractions in any position. The body position you take now should be for your comfort. Here are some of the most common positions for active labor:

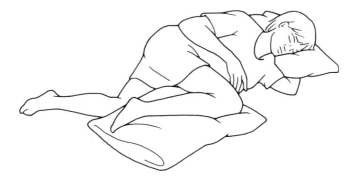

- Lying on either your right or left side.

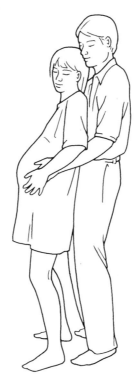

- Standing, supported by a person or leaning over a table or against the wall.

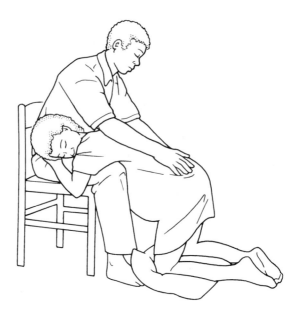

- On hands and knees on a level surface. This is especially helpful in taking any pressure from the baby's head off your back.

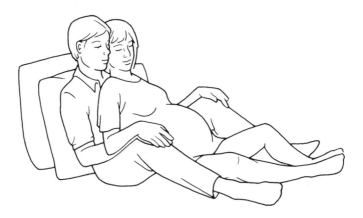

- Semi-reclining in a chair or bed. This tends to feel better than sitting directly upright because of the pressure of the baby's head.

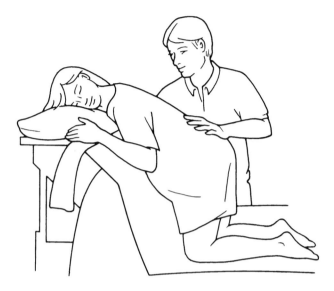

- On hands and knees, leaning against the raised head of a birthing bed. This was my favorite during my labor.

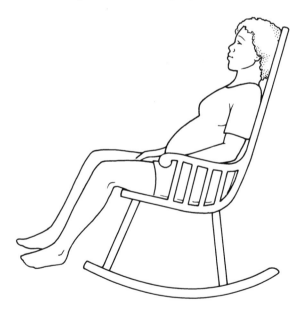

- Rocking in a rocking chair.

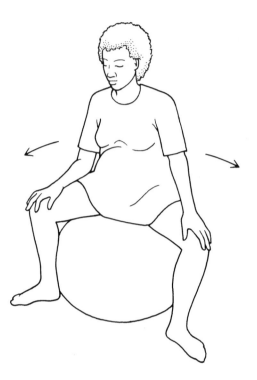

- Sitting on a birthing (exercise) ball. The flexibility of the ball and its slight bounce can make sitting on it very comfortable. The semi-squatting position helps, too; sitting on a low stool or a toilet can have a similar effect. Most birthing centers and maternity units have birthing balls.

Focus. Focusing is a way of keeping yourself centered during intense contractions. There are several ways to focus.

Close your eyes and concentrate on some image. You might visualize a soothing scene, imagine a color, or concentrate on the spots of light you see when your eyes are closed. Or you might visualize your body as a flower opening to give birth to the baby.

Look for an object or a mark on the floor or wall one to two feet away. Tell yourself you must keep your eyes on that spot throughout your entire contraction. Women who lose their focal point tend to lose their concentration, breathing, and feeling of control over the contraction.

Pay attention to the sound of your breath. Hear yourself inhale. Hear yourself exhale. Some women vocalize as they exhale.

Focus on your contraction. Mentally follow it as it begins, climbs, peaks, descends, and ends. Women who keep their focus also keep their concentration and their control over their breathing.

Breathing for labor. I often advise against trying to control the very uncontrollable experience of labor. Although you can't control contractions, you *can* control how you respond to them.

In childbirth-preparation classes, especially Lamaze, women have been taught several breathing patterns to use during labor. When I first began teaching childbirth classes in 1985, we taught seven types of breathing patterns. Over several years, I saw that even women who had learned and practiced the breathing techniques forgot the lessons completely when they came into the hospital in labor. There was simply too much to learn, too much to remember, and too much to choose from.

In all the first meetings of my PillowTalk classes, I ask the participants what they think about breathing patterns for labor. Over 75 percent say, "They don't work," "They're silly," "I'm not going to do that!" or "My friend said that with the first contraction, everything she had learned went right out the window!"

From long experience, I will tell you emphatically that learning to breathe in a controlled way is the single most important preparation you can make for labor. The breathing doesn't have to be of a certain kind—abdominal or chest, slow or fast. I have seen women breathe a hundred ways, and it works simply because they simply do it.

As I've said before, strong labor contractions can literally take your breath away. During a contraction, you are unable to walk, talk, eat, or socialize. You can react by tensing with fear, yelling, or crying. Or you can do something that truly can help make the contraction more manageable. *You can breathe in a focused way.*

We all have different ways of breathing in different circumstances. We breathe when we are anxious, when we are afraid, when we do aerobic exercise, when we do yoga. During labor, we can use the same breathing techniques that we use in other activities. The trick is to find a way of breathing that works for you. It must be your own; it must feel natural and relaxed. Some women are quiet, some make noise. Several years ago, I cared for an opera singer in labor, who—I kid you not—sang through her contractions. As long as it feels natural, whatever pattern of breathing and vocalizing you choose will be right for you.

If you do exercise such as running or yoga, I suggest starting out by breathing the same way you would during that activity. Any two women in labor may have breathing styles that are very different from one another. A runner may be comfortable breathing fast. A woman who practices yoga or meditation may find that slower, deep breaths allow her to focus more effectively. Your own comfort with how you breathe is what makes the breathing effective. Although you may alter your breathing in labor, it helps to start with a familiar pattern.

In case you do not already have a preferred type of breathing, here are two simple patterns. I could offer more, but I have learned that when women have only a couple to choose from, they are more likely to use one or more of them.

Each of these patterns starts and ends with a *cleansing breath*, that is, a breath that is full and deep. It helps you frame your contractions, allowing you to deal with them one at a time.

Slow Breathing

1. Take a cleansing breath as each contraction begins.
2. Breathe slowly and deeply, at half your normal respiration rate, and preferably in through your nose and out through your mouth.
3. Take a cleansing breath at the end of the contraction.

Modified Breathing

1. Take a cleansing breath as each contraction begins.
2. Breathe fast, at twice your normal respiration rate, and preferably in through your nose and out through your mouth.
3. Take a cleansing breath at the end of the contraction.

When I first started teaching childbirth classes, I had been taught that slow, deep breathing was very good to start with and that the modified, faster breathing was more effective as the frequency and pain of contractions increased. In practice, I haven't found this to be the case. More often, I see that women prefer to use one or the other throughout labor. It's good to be familiar with both so that you can choose between them when you encounter the pain of contractions.

Although the breathing patterns are simple, this doesn't mean that all you have to do is read these pages to know what to do in labor. Since labor is a primal physical activity, your intellect isn't going to be helping much. It can be hard to think about what you read in a book while you are in labor. You will be able to use your breathing more if you practice before labor begins.

Your practice can be very simple. Take 5 minutes a day, perhaps in the shower, on a walk, or while you are doing another simple activity.

Breathing and Visualization Practice

1. Find your focal point, or close your eyes.
2. Take your initial cleansing breath, and begin either slow or modified breathing.
3. Imagine that you are climbing up a hill, getting up to the top, and then coming back down. Visualize yourself climbing up the hill as the contraction gets stronger, reaching the top of the hill as the contraction peaks, and climbing down as the contraction fades. If your partner is with you, have him tell you about your climb and descent as he times your imaginary 1-minute contraction. Take 20 seconds or so to climb up the mountain, 10 or 15 at the top, and another 20 as you descend.

4. Finish with another deep, cleansing breath.
5. Repeat the exercise using the second breathing pattern for active labor.

This combined visualization and breathing exercise can be very helpful in preparing you for mentally managing contractions, which ascend, peak, and descend much like a mountain climb.

Tori's Tip:
Ways to Cope with Labor

Think about the day of your labor as a working day. It's not like a holiday celebration that has to follow a certain pattern. There is no use in worrying about how the day will go.

Don't go to the hospital or birth center too early. Unless your practitioner gives you different instructions, use the 5-1-1 Recipe (pages 270 and 273).

Do whatever will help you the most whenever it is most likely to help you. For early labor, distraction is the best coping tool.

Use relaxation, visualization, and breathing techniques. Some women use all these tools; others prefer only one or two. These techniques can help dramatically with active labor.

Know that labor takes on a life of its own. Although relaxation and breathing techniques can help you handle your contractions, you can't control them. Let your body follow its own rhythms.

Move around so that you can find your most comfortable position. Change positions whenever you become uncomfortable.

Ask for the kind of touch or massage you want. Light touch is soothing for some women in labor but distracting for others. Firm pressure on your lower back may be very helpful.

Since I had practiced breathing patterns in my classes for so many years, I thought I would use one of these patterns during my own labor. What had been missing in all my years of practice, though, was *pain*. When I had my own strong contractions, I buried my head in Ray's chest and said, "Ow, ow, ow, ow, ow," as though I had stubbed my toe. This was certainly a different way of coping than any I'd taught, but my breathing and vocalizing were focused and controlled, and they worked for me. Having mastered focused breathing, I was able to select a new and effective pattern when I really needed it.

Try laboring in water. Sitting in a warm bath or sitting or standing in a shower can often make a strong contraction feel entirely different and much more manageable. Your practitioner may ask you not to submerse yourself after your water bag has broken, but a shower is generally allowed anytime. Some birth centers and hospitals have large, inflatable pools that can be used in labor, and a portable one can sometimes be rented and brought in or used at home. (Except in home births, women generally don't give birth in water.)

Keep hydrated and energized. Take regular sips of cool drinks, suck on juice bars or ice, and have an occasional spoonful of honey.

Trust in your practitioner and your support people. It's really tough to have a baby all by yourself. Let others help you.

Always remember that labor lasts for a finite time. Try not to think of the hours ahead. Take your contractions one at a time. No matter how strong they are, they will generally last only about 1 minute. You can cope that long. At the end of the minute, you will get a break.

Never lose sight of why you are laboring. Keep in your mind's eye on the beautiful baby you will soon be holding in your arms.

TRANSITION PHASE

In this short phase, which lasts only 1 to 3 hours, the cervix dilates from about 7 centimeters to about 10 centimeters, its maximum diameter. Contractions come about 1½ to 2 minutes apart, peak sharply, and last as long as 90 seconds. This phase—called *transition* because it is a transition to the pushing stage—is very intense. The contractions are at their strongest. For most women, the start of the pushing stage will come as a relief.

A hallmark of transition is that the positions, breathing patterns, or other coping techniques that were helpful in active labor suddenly stop being effective. You may find it hard to get comfortable, massage may no longer be helpful, and your partner's soothing voice may soothe no more. You may feel nauseated, shaky, a bit panicky, and alternately hot and cold. You may vomit. All of this is normal.

It's very important to have your partner or another supporter as well as your labor nurse or midwife by your side at this time. Some women like to have close physical contact; others want their helpers nearby but not hovering. You may need help with each of your contractions. Deal with them one at a time. It helps to remember, or to be reminded, that each contraction will end, and you will always get a break, however brief, before the next one. It also helps to remember that your baby will soon be here.

A third breathing pattern can be very effective during transition:

Breath-Blow Breathing

1. Take a cleansing breath as each contraction begins, and relax.
2. Breathe rhythmically through your mouth. Take three short breaths in and out, and then take another breath in and a long, blowing breath out.
3. Take a cleansing breath at the end of the contraction.

Sometimes during transition, a woman feels the urge to push before her cervix is completely dilated. Your nurse or your practitioner will probably check your cervix if you feel you need to push. If your cervix is not yet fully dilated, pushing against it could cause it to become swollen and could slow its dilation. In this case, use breath-blow breathing, but blow after each inhalation.

Second Stage: Pushing

When your cervix is completely dilated, the work of pushing begins. You may not feel the urge to push immediately. It is more productive to wait until you actually feel the urge rather than to push solely because someone says your cervix is completely dilated. Pushing is hard work, and you want it to be as effective as possible. This stage usually lasts 1 to 2 hours.

The urge to push, or bear down, comes with each contraction. Contractions tend to come less frequently in the pushing stage, and this is helpful, because a longer rest period between contractions can make your efforts stronger and more productive.

The urge to push feels like being very constipated and having to have a bowel movement *now*. Some women worry that they will have an actual bowel movement while pushing. This sometimes happens. If it happens to you, the nurse, doula, or midwife or doctor won't be at all bothered by it and will take care of it immediately. In fact, since you bear down to push out a baby in the same way you do to have a bowel movement, your caregiver will give you accolades for pushing in exactly the right spot. So don't let worries about a bowel movement hold you back from pushing effectively.

Positions for pushing. Several positions are effective in helping the baby move through the pelvis and birth canal (vagina). The most common of these positions are these:

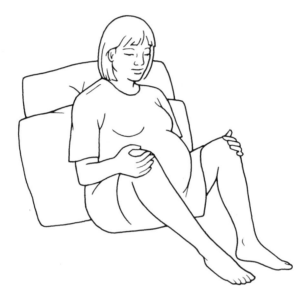

• Semi-reclining with the pelvis angled

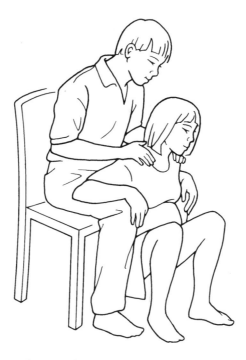

- Squatting, so that gravity assists in the downward movement of the baby

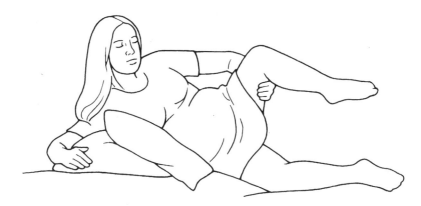

- Side-lying, while pulling your leg toward you

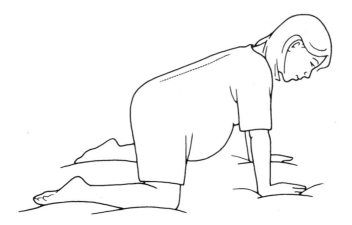

- Hands and knees, which can help rotate the baby's head into a more efficient position

The labor and birthing beds in hospitals and birth centers are designed to accommodate several positions for pushing. You can place your feet on footrests; you can place your knees over a leg support; or you can squat with the aid of a bar attached to the bed. Your nurse or midwife will help you get into the position that works best for you.

Breathing for pushing. There are two effective breathing patterns for pushing. The first works better for some women, the second for others. Your nurse, doctor, or midwife may suggest which is moving your baby most efficiently.

CONVENTIONAL PUSHING

1. Take two cleansing breaths as the urge to push builds.
2. Inhale deeply, hold your breath, and bear down for 10 seconds.
3. As you hold your breath, tighten your abdominal muscles and push the small of your back toward your partner's hand or the bed. This straightens out your lower back.
4. After 10 seconds, release your breath while keeping your abdominal muscles tight.
5. Continue this pattern for the length of the contraction.
6. Take a cleansing breath at the end of the contraction. Relax, and have a drink or an ice chip.

CONTROLLED EXHALATION, OR GENTLE PUSHING

1. Take two cleansing breaths.
2. Inhale a full breath.
3. As you tighten your abdominal muscles and flatten your back, let air slowly escape, and make a grunting sound. Grunting often comes very naturally.
4. Continue to release your breath slowly while tightening your abdominal muscles.
5. After 10 seconds, release your breath, and repeat the pattern until the contraction ends.
6. Take a cleansing breath, and relax.

Near the end of your pushing stage, your practitioner will guide you in easing the baby out. As your baby's head stretches your perineum, you will feel a hot, burning sensation, commonly known as the "ring of fire." This is generally indicative of the last push before the baby is born.

What Is an Episiotomy?

An incision made in the perineum from the vagina toward the anus, an episiotomy is done when a baby's delivery must be hurried or when significant perineal tearing is likely to occur during a birth. As is well documented, an episiotomy does not prevent minor tearing, is no easier to repair than a natural tear, and does not prevent uterine prolapse. Allowing the perineum to stretch slowly and applying oil and massage to the perineum *does* help prevent a tear. A minor tear is preferable to an episiotomy. Today, episiotomies are *not* routinely done.

Third Stage: Birth of the Placenta

As soon as your baby is born, provided the two of you are doing well, you or your practitioner will bring the baby up to your chest. This is a wonderful, magical moment, when all your hard work is finally rewarded. It is a time like no other.

While you hold your baby, your practitioner will await the release of the placenta from the wall of your uterus. First, the umbilical cord will come loose, and then there will be a small increase in vaginal bleeding. Your doctor or midwife will ask you to push gently, and the placenta will pass. This will probably happen 5 to 20 minutes after the baby's birth. The passage of the placenta is usually not uncomfortable.

It is very uncommon for the placenta not to pass properly. If this happens, the practitioner manually removes it.

Your practitioner will press your belly to be sure your uterus has contracted to the size and firmness of a grapefruit. If necessary, the nurse or practitioner may massage your uterus until it becomes firm. The uterus must remain firm to prevent excessive bleeding from the site where the placenta was attached to the wall of your uterus.

A Little about Labor-and-Delivery Nurses

Some popular books on childbirth leave a huge void concerning the support provided by labor-and-delivery nurses (also called perinatal, maternity, or maternal-child nurses). I am troubled that nurses are either not mentioned at all or are referred to as "overworked medical personnel." Nurses can be busy, and hospitals are often far from being homey. But the suggestion that nurses have neither the time nor the ability to care for all the needs of a woman giving birth is simply wrong. Having been a perinatal nurse for over 20 years, I can tell you that maternity nurses provide a high level of physical, emotional, and often spiritual care to laboring women and their families.

Presume that you will be cared for in your hospital or birth center by kind, intelligent, and compassionate people. If you needed knee surgery, you wouldn't expect incompetent and uncompassionate care. Why would you when you are planning something as wonderful as having a baby? How unfair it is to set up this expectation.

Maternity units today are designed to be welcoming, aesthetically pleasing, and as homelike as possible. At San Francisco's California Pacific Medical Center, where over 500 babies are born each month, every woman in active labor has one-on-one nursing support. There are no mandatory IVs for normal labor, no enemas, and no separation of mom and baby unless needed for the health or safety of one or both. Fetal monitoring can be intermittent, and episiotomies are not routine. Moms are welcome to walk in labor, eat lightly, and have anyone they want at the birth. Whether a woman chooses to have her baby in a quiet, dimly lit room without medication, or with an epidural and a camera, she is cared for with skill, sensitivity, and kindness. Nationwide, many small community hospitals and large urban medical centers are adopting this style of care. Tour your hospital or birth center for a better sense of what your experience will be like. Some tours are given by nurses, who can answer questions about policies and procedures. If the tour is led by a volunteer, save specific questions about your care for your practitioner.

Fourth Stage: Immediate Postpartum

During the first 2 hours after birth, you will be able to rest, eat and drink, breastfeed your baby, and simply take in your amazing baby and the experience you have just had. Your care providers, meanwhile, will make sure that you are recovering well.

A baby is normally quite awake during this time. Soon after the birth, the baby will express his interest in breastfeeding by *rooting* turning his face toward your breast and moving his tongue and mouth. Breastfeeding releases oxytocin, which helps keep the uterus well contracted. In the first few days after birth, this release of oxytocin can cause strong uterine cramping during breastfeeding.

We'll discuss breastfeeding and your newborn baby more in the next chapter.

Support in Labor

Your job on the day that you are in labor is to labor and give birth to your child. That's all, and that's plenty. Everything else is the job of your supporters. Good support throughout your labor will be your best coping tool. This support can be provided by your partner, another family member or close friend or two, a labor nurse, a doula (page 249), your midwife or doctor, or any combination of these. Their job is to help keep you calm, comfortable, and well hydrated, and to encourage and reassure you throughout labor. Over the centuries, what has helped laboring women the most has been the constant presence, reassurance, and practical aid of others around them. This is still true today.

If you currently lack strong trust in the people who will care for you, change your plans if you can. If you aren't sure your partner will be sufficiently supportive when you are in labor, ask a close friend to be there as well. Having another support person with you might make a big difference.

Keep in mind, though, that you don't want an audience. Plan to have with you in labor only people who will give you emotional support and practical help. It may seem like a nice idea now to have someone attend your birth as an observer, but when you are actually in labor, you might wish this person were somewhere else. If you are going to ask any extra family member or friend to be with you, you might add that you may change your mind once you are in labor. Talking about this possibility in advance could prevent hurt feelings on the big day.

It can be particularly difficult to have a child with you in labor. If a child does attend the birth, it's important to have an adult who is specifically responsible for caring for the child. This will allow you and your partner to fully focus on your labor.

Medications and Medical Procedures

Today you can choose to relieve your labor pains with relaxation and focused breathing, analgesia (page 296), epidural anesthesia (page 298), or any combination of these. Medications and medical procedures can affect your labor, but this doesn't necessarily mean that the effect will be detrimental. For example, epidural anesthesia might prolong your labor for an hour, but the relief from pain may make the experience more positive for you.

To your care providers, the health and safety of you and your baby are of the utmost concern. Vast numbers of studies are conducted before a drug or a medical procedure is sanctioned for use in labor. Today's medications and medical procedures for labor, when prescribed and used appropriately, have been found to be safe for both moms and babies.

ANALGESIA

This is pain relief without the loss of other sensations. Analgesics are used today to relieve all types of pain. These drugs range from mild pain relievers such as acetaminophen (Tylenol is the best-known brand) to potent opioids, such as morphine. Among the analgesics used in labor are the narcotics morphine, fentanyl, Nubain, and Stadol. Practitioners in different parts of the country tend to have different preferences for these drugs and their combinations, but all these medications provide essentially the same type of pain relief, although the onset and duration of relief vary somewhat. Medications for labor are generally given either as an intramuscular injection or intravenously.

The medication takes effect shortly after it is given, by decreasing the intensity of the pain you feel. In other words, you can still feel the contraction, but the drug "takes the edge off' the pain or "smoothes over the peak" of the contraction. You may want to continue to use focused breathing and relaxation after taking the medication, but you will probably feel better able to cope with your contractions and more relaxed between them.

Unlike some medications used in labor as recently as the mid-1980s, today's medications don't make a woman feel extremely sedated, or "drugged." A narcotic can cause some initial dizziness, but this generally passes very quickly.

The pain relief from a narcotic generally lasts from 1 to 4 hours, and the dose can usually be repeated if you are still in early or active labor. If a narcotic were at its peak effect at the time of birth, the drug would lessen the baby's reflexes to cough, take deep breaths, clear her lungs, and breastfeed. For this reason, practitioners are careful not to administer narcotics immediately before a baby's birth. When the medication is given earlier in labor, the baby has time to metabolize and eliminate most of it from her system. In the past 25 years, I have seen little or no difference among the behaviors of babies born to moms who had no medication, moms who had analgesia, and moms who had epidural anesthesia.

NITROUS OXIDE (N$_2$O)

You've probably heard of, or even experienced, nitrous oxide (laughing gas) during a dental procedure. Although in the US this is what we primarily use it for, in Europe and Australia it is also used to manage labor pain. In recent years, it has gained popularity in this country, and more and more hospitals now offer it.

The laboring mom has a hand-held mask by her bedside, through which she can breathe the gas in when she is feeling pain or a contraction, temporarily feeling relief. When she removes the mask and exhales, the gas dissipates. Because it is expelled from the mom's system quickly, it doesn't cross the placenta. Women often say they like it because they feel more in control of their pain relief.

ANESTHESIA

The goal of anesthesia is complete pain relief. There are three types of anesthesia: general, regional, and local.

With *general anesthesia*, a drug is either inhaled as a gas or injected intravenously. The medication causes you to lose consciousness for a time. General anesthesia is not used routinely in labor, because it can depress respiration in the newborn. Since the medication can be given very quickly, however, general anesthesia is used in emergency cesareans, when the baby must be born without delay. Once general anesthesia has been given, the baby is delivered as soon as possible to minimize the amount of anesthetic that reaches him.

Regional anesthesia provides relief from pain in a specific area of your body. For labor and for cesarean birth, anesthetic medication is injected into the lumbar region (lower middle part) of your back. The nerve roots traveling from this area to the rest of the body are bathed in the anesthetic, and as a result, you lose pain and all sensation from your waist down to your feet (or, for a cesarean birth, from your nipple line down to your toes).

There are two types of regional anesthesia, spinal and epidural. An anesthesiologist or a nurse-anesthetist performs both. Both types of anesthesia are administered when the woman is sitting up with rounded shoulders or lying on her side.

Spinal anesthesia is used primarily for scheduled cesarean births. A single injection of numbing medication (in the "-caine" family of drugs) is given directly through the spinal membrane, into the fluid-filled sac that surrounds your spinal cord. As you can see from the illustrations (page 299), the needle does not pass close to the spinal cord. A spinal anesthetic takes effect within a few minutes, and the effect lasts for approximately 2 hours. Because the period of pain relief is so short, spinal anesthesia is not used for labor. (For more about spinals, see page 314.)

More useful for labor is *epidural anesthesia*. The medication is essentially the same but with a different combination of lidocaine-type drugs. It is also a narcotic. The site of the injection is slightly different from that of a spinal. With an epidural, the medication is injected into a hollow area between the vertebrae and the spinal cord, directly outside (*epi*) the sac (*dura*) where the spinal fluid is located. The medication then flows across the spinal membrane. After the initial injection is given, a small, flexible catheter is placed into the epidural space. With this catheter in place, the woman can receive more medication anytime during labor. Sometimes, an infusion pump is also attached, and a continuous drip of medication (similar to an IV) is started. The procedure takes 10 to 30 minutes to complete. The anesthetic takes effect more slowly than with a spinal, about 20 minutes for full relief. Then you will probably no longer feel contractions, although you may feel some pressure, which can be helpful when it is time to push.

You may have heard of something called a *walking* or an *in-trathecal epidural*, in which narcotic only is injected into the epidural space, without anesthetic. The procedure is called a *walking epidural* because the legs do not become numb and the mother can walk around comfortably for a time afterward. This can be helpful for women who wish to be up for as long as possible yet still want pain relief. Studies have shown, though, that the majority of women who choose a walking epidural ultimately move on to a standard epidural, which numbs the lower body and therefore prevents any walking.

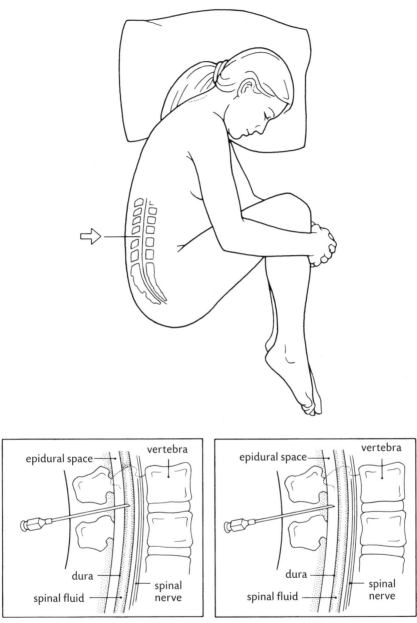

epidural space

vertebra

dura

spinal fluid

spinal nerve

Spinal Block

epidural space

vertebra

dura

spinal fluid

spinal nerve

Epidural Block

Although epidural anesthesia is safe, the medical procedure does have side effects and so requires a higher level of monitoring. Here are some important things to know about epidurals:

- The most common side effect is lowered blood pressure. To maintain your blood pressure, you will be given fluids intravenously, and your blood pressure will be monitored closely with an automatic monitoring cuff.
- Because an epidural erases sensation from waist to toes, you probably won't feel when you need to pee. If your bladder becomes full, you may have a urinary catheter placed in your bladder.
- Although you may be able to move in bed, your legs will not support your body, so you will have to remain in bed until the baby is born.
- Although it had been previously thought that epidural anesthesia could slow labor, especially if the anesthesia was given before the onset of active labor, current research shows that there is no significant increase in the lengths of labor in women who choose to have epidural anesthesia.
- Pain relief may vary. Over 90 percent of women experience total pain relief from an epidural, but a small percentage experience partial relief or none at all. Sometimes the procedure must be repeated to provide full relief.
- A small percentage of women experience increased temperature, itching, or both as a side effect of the medication. The symptoms are generally mild, and they can be treated if necessary with an antihistamine.
- In about 4 percent of cases, a small amount of spinal fluid leaks from the puncture site. This can cause a severe headache, which is treated by injecting a small amount of the mother's blood into the space.
- In general, women who have an epidural push very well with guidance and support. It is not necessarily likely that there would be an increased chance of having an assisted delivery (page 304), with forceps or a vacuum extractor.

- The drugs used in epidural anesthesia cross the placenta. These drugs have been well studied, however, and are considered safe for the baby.
- As with any medications or medical procedures, there are risks of rare complications. With an epidural, these risks include reaction to the medication, infection, paralysis, and nerve damage. The rate of these complications ranges from 1 in 50,000, to 1 in 250,000 or more.

There is much ongoing discussion about whether having epidural anesthesia increases the likelihood of having a cesarean birth. Some years ago, several retrospective studies found that women who had epidurals were as much as three times more likely than other women to have cesarean sections. As researchers have continued to review and analyze hospital records, however, these findings have been disputed. According to the National Institute of Child Health and Human Development, epidural anesthesia alone does not appear to increase a woman's chances of having a cesarean birth. More research is being conducted in this area.

Local anesthesia blocks pain in just one area of your body. The most common use is in dental work. During childbirth, local anesthesia may be used to numb the vagina and perineum during repair of a perineal tear or during an episiotomy (page 292).

Get Pain Relief without Drugs

Alternative methods of pain relief that women have found helpful in labor include hypnosis, acupuncture, and transcutaneous electrical nerve stimulation (TENS). TENS applies electrical impulses to your lower back to diminish awareness of pain. You may wish to investigate whether these options are available in your own community.

FETAL MONITORING

A nurse or midwife monitors the baby's heart rate to ensure the baby's well-being during labor. Changes in the rate may indicate whether the baby is getting enough oxygen.

The baby's heart rate can be monitored in various ways:

- A *fetoscope* is a manual stethoscope specifically designed to listen to the heartbeat of a baby in the womb.
- A *Doppler listening device* is a small, hand-held ultrasound monitor.
- *Electronic fetal monitoring (EFM)* keeps an ongoing record of the baby's heart rate.

In hospitals, most babies are monitored with external EFM. A flat ultrasound device is placed on your abdomen over the area of your baby's heart. You are generally not restricted to bed; you can sit in a chair, stand, or squat as you wish. The monitor connects to a small computer placed next to the birthing bed. This computer is often connected to a larger one so that nurses can observe the heart-rate patterns on a screen outside your room.

Telemetry monitoring is now widely available. With telemetry, the electronic fetal monitor device doesn't have to be plugged into the computer. You can walk and even take a shower or bath during telemetry monitoring.

During labor, a baby's heart normally beats between 110 and 160 times per minute. Variations are usually normal and healthy, but atypical changes may cause your practitioner to be concerned. As long as your baby is demonstrating normal heart-rate variations and is thus judged to be tolerating labor well, and as long as you haven't received a narcotic, anesthesia, or oxytocin (page 311), monitoring will be intermittent. Otherwise, EFM will be used continuously.

If your practitioner is concerned about your baby's heart-rate pattern or is unable to monitor it adequately with external EFM, he or she may put an *internal fetal scalp electrode* into your vagina and attach it directly to the baby's head. Internal monitoring can provide more detailed information about your baby's well-being.

Occasionally, continuous fetal monitoring falsely indicates that a baby is in *fetal distress*, or not getting enough oxygen. This can result in unnecessary medical interventions. If your practitioner judges from the EFM tracing that your baby is in distress, ask questions about anything you don't understand. You can and should be part of the decisions regarding what happens next.

UTERINE MONITORING

With EFM, the frequency and duration of uterine contractions can be followed with another small electronic device called a *toco-dynamometer* or *toco* for short. This is a pressure-sensing monitor that detects the tightening of your uterus during a contraction. It doesn't measure the strength of contractions, but it indicates when contractions begin and end and how long they last. The monitor is plugged into the same computer that the fetal monitor is connected to. Like EFM, uterine monitoring can be done intermittently or continuously.

If your practitioner suspects that your contractions are too weak to dilate your cervix, he or she can measure their strength by placing an internal-pressure monitor called an *intrauterine pressure catheter (IUPC)* inside your uterus.

An IUPC might also be used if the baby's heart-rate pattern shows signs that her umbilical cord is being compressed during contractions. Compression of the umbilical cord could be caused by decreased amniotic fluid around the baby. Placing an IUPC allows saline fluid to be flushed into your uterus, and the additional fluid can help to "float" the baby's umbilical cord. This procedure, called an *amnioinfusion*, can also be done to reduce the concentration of meconium (page 266) in the amniotic fluid.

ASSISTED DELIVERY

Sometimes a baby needs to be delivered more quickly than a mother is able to push him out. Usually this is because the baby's heart rate has slowed. Assisted delivery can also be necessary when a woman is exhausted and unable to continue pushing, and it can be used to turn a baby who is in a difficult, *posterior* position (page 274), facing the same way as the mother. In such cases, provided the cervix is completely dilated and the baby is low in the birth canal, the doctor may recommend the use of either forceps or a vacuum extractor. *Forceps* are smooth, metal instruments, shaped like curved salad tongs, that are carefully applied to the sides of the baby's head. A *vacuum extractor* is a plastic cup placed on the baby's head and attached to a suction device. The choice between the two may depend on which the doctor has been trained to use or which is the most appropriate in the particular situation. Assisted delivery, with either forceps or vacuum extraction, is used in about 10 percent of births.

Assisted delivery is usually undertaken after a mother has been pushing for some time. During a contraction and while the mother is pushing, the doctor applies controlled traction and guides the baby through the birth canal. The doctor does not pull the baby out and will not use either of these methods if he or she feels that the baby is too large to deliver vaginally.

CESAREAN SECTION

Most of the time, a vaginal birth is preferable to a cesarean birth. In several situations, however, a cesarean may be the safest way to deliver a baby:

Breech or transverse position of the baby. Instead of being in a vertex, or head-down, position, the baby may have her bottom or feet down or may be lying horizontally. To avoid the possibility that the baby's head will become trapped inside the uterus, the vast majority of breech babies today are delivered by cesarean section. If a woman is going to try for a vaginal delivery of a breech baby, the baby needs to be of average or smaller size, as measured by ultrasound, the mother's pelvis must measure adequately large by pelvimetry (X-ray), and the baby

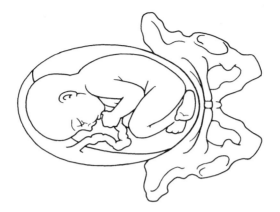

Breech Position

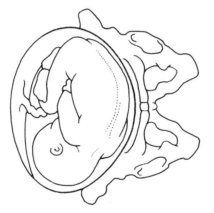

Transverse Position

must be in either a *frank* (bottom down, legs up) or *complete* (sitting) breech position. Babies who are in either a footling (one foot down), a double footling (both feet down), or a transverse (horizontal) position are only delivered by cesarean section, because of the risk of a prolapsed umbilical cord.

Prolapsed cord. This occurs when the umbilical cord moves ahead of the baby into the vagina. The cord may prolapse after the membranes rupture if the baby is in a breech or transverse position or his head is not well engaged in the mom's pelvis. This is an emergency: An immediate cesarean birth is necessary to prevent the presenting part (head, bottom, or foot) from compressing the cord and cutting off the baby's oxygen supply.

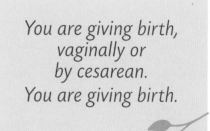

You are giving birth, vaginally or by cesarean. You are giving birth.

Twins or triplets. As discussed on page 190, the size and position of the babies may determine that a cesarean is safer.

Cephalopelvic disproportion (CPD). This occurs when the baby's head won't fit through the mother's pelvis. Typically, the problem is identified only after the mother has been in labor for some time. Either the cervix stops dilating or the baby will not descend in the pelvis, even with adequate contractions and good pushing efforts. A prolonged labor or a delayed start of labor after the rupture of the membranes may also be an indication of CPD.

Placenta previa (page 196). If the placenta completely covers the cervix, a cesarean birth is necessary. It would be dangerous for both mother and baby if the placenta were to deliver first.

Fetal distress. A cesarean may be performed to speed birth if an abnormal heart-rate pattern indicates that the baby is not receiving enough oxygen.

Placental abruption. If the placenta partially or completely separates from the uterine wall before the baby is born, the mother may hemorrhage, and the baby may lose part or all of her oxygen supply. This is an emergency: An immediate cesarean is necessary.

In the United States today, approximately 32 percent of babies are born by cesarean section. This high rate is quite controversial. Some of the reasons for it are these:

- The percentage of women who deliver vaginally after having had a prior cesarean birth has dropped sharply in recent years, in spite of the fact that 75 percent of women who attempt VBAC (vaginal birth after cesarean, page 220) succeed.
- Advances in reproductive technology have enabled women with "high-risk" conditions to become pregnant. High blood pressure, diabetes, advanced maternal age, and obesity all increase the likelihood of a cesarean birth.
- Physicians worry about malpractice lawsuits. If a baby born by vaginal delivery is injured or dies during childbirth, the physician is likely to be held liable, even if a cesarean section would not have made any difference. No other country puts such blame solely on the doctor.

A newer, more disturbing trend that has gained popularity in other countries has surfaced here in the United States recently. A woman may request a cesarean section with no medical indication at all. Her reasons may vary: She may choose a cesarean for convenience, out of fear of labor pain, or even to preserve her perineum. She may not be aware of the risks of major abdominal surgery—infection, bleeding, scarring, and a long recovery period. Many physicians will not agree to elective cesarean for a first baby, but the practice is likely to increase over the next several years.

How can you avoid an unnecessary cesarean? I suggest asking your doctor or midwife about his or her philosophy regarding cesarean birth. Ask also about the rate of cesareans among your practitioner's clients. Using a doctor, midwife, or hospital with a low cesarean rate can lessen your chance of an avoidable surgery. Making sure you'll have good support in labor is also important. One-on-one labor support has been shown to reduce the need for cesarean delivery.

When Things Don't Go As Planned

My colleagues and I joke that obstetrical nurses and doctors seem to have the worst labor stories. I'd like to share with you my own experience with severe preeclampsia, not to scare you, but to illuminate how unpredictable birth can be and to emphasize that what is most important, in the end, is a healthy mom and baby.

I was healthy, healthy, healthy, during my pregnancy. But when I arrived at the hospital in labor, my blood pressure was extremely high, 180/120. My normal blood pressure is about 90/60. I had also gained 9 pounds (4 kg) since the previous day. I was developing something called HELLP (hemolysis, elevated liver enzyme levels, and a low platelet count) syndrome, the most severe complication of preeclampsia. HELLP involves blood cells, the liver, and the kidneys and is quite unusual; only 0.5 percent of pregnant women develop it. That it had come on so suddenly meant it was especially serious.

I was quickly given medication to lower my blood pressure and to prevent seizures. I remember very little as I rapidly became sicker. Treatment for this disease is birth, but I was too ill to continue with labor. Alexander was born by cesarean section at 9:40 p.m.

INDUCTION OF LABOR

Imagine that you have passed your due date by a week or more. Your family and friends are calling to ask you if you have had the baby (as if you would have forgotten to tell them!) or, worse, why you *haven't* yet had the baby. You are more than ready for labor to begin!

There are several reasons why you might need to have an induction. The most common are these:

- Your pregnancy has gone past your due date. Current studies show that, depending on your age, it is best not to go past 40 to 41 weeks gestation. Your placenta may not be functioning as effectively and your risk of cesarean birth is higher.

I do not remember anything before noon the next day. When I look at photographs of myself holding and breast-feeding Alexander, I can barely recognize my swollen face. We went home from the hospital five days later. I lost 30 pounds (13.6 kg) in fluid over the next week.

I had thought that I'd mapped out all the possible ways my labor could go, and this one had never even occurred to me. My labor actually was fun in the beginning, but then things changed for the worse. And that happens. Not often, but sometimes.

Because I was so ill, I had a scary labor and a cesarean section; I didn't hold Alexander right after he was born; I didn't breastfeed him until 6 hours later; and I ended up staying in the hospital for five days. None of this is what I had wished for. Still, I am grateful and happy that I have a healthy, thriving son who has a healthy mom. I breastfed Alexander for a year, and we are very close. I would go through it all again to have a child like him.

Giving birth is an amazing experience, whether it happens at home with a midwife, in a hospital with an epidural, or by cesarean section. Childbirth is not an end unto itself, but rather the beginning of an incredible life.

- Your baby is growing very large, even if you haven't reached your due date, and your doctor fears that if the pregnancy continues, the baby may be too large for you to deliver vaginally.
- You have a medical condition such as high blood pressure, pre-eclampsia, or diabetes, and the condition is worsening.
- Your water bags breaks, but you do not go into labor.
- Your baby is not growing adequately and will be safer growing outside the womb. *Intrauterine growth retardation* can be caused by a variety of conditions.
- The amount of amniotic fluid around the baby is low, even though your membranes haven't ruptured.

There is a growing trend in the United States to induce labor for no medical reason at all. In fact, *elective induction* has become one of the most commonly performed medical procedures in the United States; as many as 30 percent of all inductions in this country are elective. Your practitioner will discuss the pros and cons of this with you. An elective induction cannot be done prior to 39 weeks, as there is a risk of the baby being born with respiratory problems due to incomplete lung development.

A physician can induce labor by "stripping" or tearing the membranes, by placing a synthetic prostaglandin in the cervix, by inflating a small balloon in the cervix, or by administering oxytocin intravenously.

Stripping of the membranes. Your practitioner may insert a finger through your cervix and manually separate your amniotic membranes (water bag) from the lower part of your uterus. This causes the release of prostaglandins that can sometimes initiate labor. Stripping of the membranes is often the first induction method tried.

Artificial rupture of membranes. If your cervix is "ripe" (soft and effacing) and dilated a bit, your body is quite ready for labor and perhaps just needs a jump-start. In this case, your practitioner can use a small hook to snag and break the water bag, which releases the amniotic fluid. This procedure is generally painless. Prostaglandins released in the amniotic fluid can stimulate the start of labor. Your baby's heart rate and your uterine contractions will be monitored for a period after the procedure. If contractions do not start within several hours, you may receive oxytocin.

Cervical ripening. To stimulate the softening and effacing of the cervix, physicians often use misoprostol (Cytotec), a synthetic prostaglandin used off-label for labor induction in the United States but marketed for this purpose in other parts of the world. A small tablet is taken orally several hours apart until the cervix is softened. Misoprostol occasionally initiates contractions on its own.

Foley catheter. The practitioner may insert into your cervix a catheter with a very small, uninflated balloon at the end. The balloon is then filled with a small amount of water. This puts pressure on the cervix, and the pressure stimulates the release of prostaglandins. As the cervix dilates, the balloon falls out, and the catheter is removed.

Oxytocin (Pitocin). The administration of Pitocin, a synthetic form of the natural hormone oxytocin, is the most common method of inducing labor. Pitocin, which causes uterine contractions, is given in intravenous fluid. The doses are very small at first. Over the course of several hours or a day, the amount of Pitocin is gradually increased, just as a woman's production of natural oxytocin increases as labor begins. Besides causing contractions, Pitocin stimulates the body to produce its own oxytocin.

The chance of a successful induction is much higher if the cervix is soft and partly effaced before Pitocin is given. This is why a synthetic prostaglandin is often administered first. If labor does not begin after a full day of Pitocin, the drip may be stopped and restarted the following day. Most inductions are successful by the end of the second day.

When you are receiving Pitocin, your baby's heart rate and your uterine contractions are monitored continuously. You may be able to sit in a chair rather than lie in a bed. If you have telemetry monitoring (page 302), you can walk and move about.

Pitocin doesn't take effect suddenly or dramatically; it takes time for the body to respond. You might actually be a bit bored for a few hours after a Pitocin drip has been started. To help pass the time before active labor begins, it is a good idea to have with you a book or magazine, a deck of cards, a board game, or visitors.

Pitocin can also be used after labor has begun, if the contractions are too slow or weak to dilate the cervix. The administration of Pitocin during labor is called *augmenting* labor.

You may have heard that Pitocin makes labor more difficult. This isn't necessarily so. By working together with natural oxytocin, however, Pitocin helps make labor more efficient. A more efficient labor is generally shorter, and a shorter labor is more intense.

I sometimes hear a woman say, "I was doing okay in labor, but then I got Pitocin and the contractions became horrible." In this case, she had probably been in labor so long that her uterus had become fatigued.

Either her contractions had slowed, or they were not strong enough to further dilate her cervix. She may have handled them well because they were mild. Once she got Pitocin, she had stronger contractions and her cervix began dilating more. Her contractions were more difficult because labor was progressing; the Pitocin had served its purpose.

Home methods for inducing labor. Lovemaking, orgasm, spicy foods, castor oil, herbs, and other methods seem to get labor going for some women, but for many moms, the methods haven't worked. As with Pitocin, the body must be ready to go into labor. It is difficult to push Mother Nature if she isn't ready!

Nipple stimulation is frequently recommended for either inducing or augmenting labor. When the nipples are gently rubbed, pulled, or twisted, natural oxytocin is released. But sometimes the body releases too much oxytocin, and the result is extremely prolonged contractions, lasting 2 to 5 minutes. Such long contractions can cause fetal distress (page 306). If you're tempted to use nipple stimulation to avoid a medical induction, I encourage you to discuss this with your practitioner.

Ask Tori, R.N.

WHEN THE BABY DROPS
Hi, Tori,

How will I know when the baby "drops"? Will labor start right away afterward?

—Ashley, Washington, D.C.

Ashley,

The common term for this event, *lightening*, doesn't quite convey what actually happens: The baby's head descends into the pelvis. Because of decreased pressure on the diaphragm and stomach, you will indeed feel "lightened" when your baby drops, and your breathing and digestion will become easier. You'll probably also feel the need to urinate more often, however, and you may feel pressure or aches and pains in your pelvic joints and perineum (page 150). You'll notice a change in the shape of your abdomen; the bulge will have shifted down and forward.

If this is your first baby, lightening may occur about two weeks before labor starts. In women who have given birth before, the baby often doesn't drop until labor begins.

CARPAL TUNNEL SYNDROME
Dear Tori,

Lately I've been having a burning feeling and numbness in my hands. These sensations are starting to wake me up during the night. Is this something serious?

—Michelle, New York

Dear Michelle,

You may be having symptoms of *carpal tunnel syndrome*. Although this condition occurs most commonly in women between 40 and 60 years old, often as a result of repetitive movements of the wrists and hands, it also occurs in as many as 25 percent of pregnant women.

In pregnancy, hormonal effects, swelling, and weight gain can compress the nerve inside the carpal tunnel, which is a sheath of tissue surrounding the median nerve. This nerve supplies the thumb, the first two fingers, and half of the ring finger. The symptoms of carpal tunnel syndrome are numbness, tingling, pain, and often a burning sensation in these areas, on one or both hands. Treatment includes wearing a wrist splint at night and during activities that make the symptoms worse, such as driving a car or holding a book. You may also be able to relieve the discomfort by rubbing or shaking your hands. Although the symptoms of carpal tunnel syndrome can be disturbing, they almost always disappear after the baby is born.

THE SAFETY OF SPINAL ANESTHESIA

Dear Tori,

I am pregnant with my second child. My first child was born by cesarean section under general anesthesia because of fetal distress. For this second baby, I will be having another cesarean, but my doctor told me that he would rather I have a spinal anesthetic than go to sleep. My question is this: Are there any side effects from a spinal? The thought of a needle going near my spine is quite scary!

—Allison, South Dakota

Dear Allison,

Except in emergencies, spinal anesthesia is usually preferred over general anesthesia for cesarean births. General anesthesia has no long-term effects on babies, but if they are exposed to it in the uterus for more than a few minutes, they can be quite sleepy at birth. Spinal anesthesia works quickly and lasts for only a couple of hours. It is very safe for the baby.

The thought of a needle in the back can be frightening. I hope that by explaining the process of spinal anesthesia, I can ease your fears about it.

An anesthesiologist administers a spinal anesthetic by placing a specially designed needle through the membrane outside your spinal fluid in the lumbar region of your back (well below the end of your spinal cord.) The doctor injects a numbing medication directly into the spinal fluid.

A spinal differs from an epidural in that, with a spinal, the needle passes through the membrane where the spinal fluid is; with an epidural, it does not. Also, with an epidural a tiny catheter is inserted. This allows more doses to be given for longer pain relief. Both procedures produce numbing from the breasts or belly button down to your toes.

Fewer than 4 percent of women who have spinal anesthesia get a "spinal headache," which occurs after a small amount of spinal fluid leaks out. This problem is corrected with a "blood patch," in which a small amount of the woman's own blood is injected into the area.

BLUE COHOSH FOR INDUCTION OF LABOR

Dear Tori,

I read about an herb called blue cohosh, which can induce labor contractions. Do you have any information on this? Is it harmful for the baby? I am 41 weeks pregnant and would like to try some natural method of induction. Thanks.

—Libby, Rhode Island

Dear Libby,

Blue cohosh, or *Caulophyllum thalictroides*, is also sometimes called blueberry root, papoose root, squawroot, yellow ginseng, blue ginseng, or beech drops. Harvested in wooded areas of eastern North America, the root was originally used by Native Americans as a uterine stimulant. It is used in various forms to induce labor contractions. In my experience, blue cohosh can indeed cause uterine contractions, but it does not necessarily initiate labor. It can also have the unpleasant side effects of diarrhea, nausea, vomiting, and abdominal cramping.

Like other medicines, herbal remedies can be very powerful. It is very important to talk with your midwife or doctor before taking any medicinal herb.

WAITING FOR THE BABY

Hi, Tori,

Aarrgg! I am 38 weeks along and losing my mind! Do you have any tips for how I can get through this waiting? I am so excited I can't stand it!

—Jocelyn, Hawaii

Dear Jocelyn,

Women everywhere understand how you feel. I have some ideas for you. They are simple, and they come from the experts, women like you who have been waiting, waiting, waiting. Enjoy this quiet time before your baby's birth!

- Visit a new or elegant restaurant.
- Catch up on the latest movies, or enjoy old classics.
- Enjoy a walk, every day.
- Swim.
- Make a couple of stews or casseroles, and freeze them for after the baby is born.
- Have lunch with a friend.
- Treat yourself to a massage.
- Make a list of numbers to call when the baby is born.
- Spend a romantic night or weekend in a hotel with your partner.
- Take a bubble bath.
- Shop for yourself, not the baby.
- Buy some fresh flowers.
- Bake cookies or bread.

- Visit a local museum.
- Read a good book that's not about birth or babies.
- Write a letter to someone you don't see often enough.
- Go to a concert.
- Go dancing with your partner.
- Play with your pet, as it may sense that change is coming.
- Ask your mate for a foot rub.
- Go to the beach.
- Spend an evening cuddling in front of a fire with your sweetie.
- Have your partner take some sexy and silly photos of your pregnant body.
- Look at your baby pictures and your partner's.
- Savor being two before you become three!

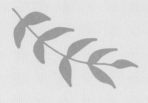

DAD'S CORNER

Your mate may be in nesting mode now and may have become very particular about her physical environment. The physical side of your relationship may have mellowed into holding and cuddling, although some couples experience a resurgence of sensuality in these last few weeks. If your mate is on bed rest, she is by now an expert on cabin fever and may require some extra pampering to maintain her equilibrium. She needs as much fresh air as possible. She'll enjoy funny and romantic movies, but avoid programs about war or politics. Pregnant women aren't fragile or helpless, but bringing a new life into being makes a person very sensitive about the state of the world.

Your Role in Labor. You may be feeling uncertain of what you'll be doing while your partner is in labor. Your very presence will mean much to her. When I say presence, I mean that with words or actions or both, you convey to her that you are with her, all the way. You are not on the sidelines; you are beside her, providing encouragement, support, and reassurance.

You may be planning to be her sole moral supporter during labor and birth, and such intimacy can be a wonderful thing. Or the two of you may choose to have a friend, relative, or doula with you to provide comfort and reassurance. If you aren't comfortable providing all the moral support for your partner, planning for a helper may be a good idea. Women who have constant support in labor generally have shorter labors, describe their labors as being more manageable, and have birth experiences that are more positive.

There are many ways you will support your partner. Here are some especially helpful things that you can do for her:

- Assist her in maintaining a relaxed body and attitude. Help her to be as loose and limp as possible.
- Encourage her to walk and to change positions frequently. Alternate walking with rest periods.
- In early (latent) labor, help distract her from her contractions. Walk in the park, go to a movie, or even go shopping.

- Encourage her to drink liquids frequently.
- Talk to her softly and lovingly during her contractions. If each of her contractions lasts about the same length of time, use your watch to let her know when she is halfway done. If she is on a uterine monitor, you can tell when the contraction is starting, peaking, and ending by watching the tracing on paper. Knowing that a contraction is nearly over can help her get through it.
- Help her with her breathing techniques and concentration.
- Remind her to deal with just one contraction at a time.
- Encourage and assist her to shower or bathe. It is wonderful to labor in water!
- Touch and support her physically during each contraction, unless she prefers not to be touched.
- Massage her wherever it feels good to her. Apply counterpressure on her lower back. To protect your own back, position yourself close to her, lean in, and use your body weight rather than arm strength to apply pressure.
- *Occasionally* time and record contractions.
- Apply balm to her lips if they are getting dry.
- Praise her often. Remain positive, especially if her confidence is dwindling. Don't let her lose sight of the fact that she will have a baby in her arms soon.
- Offer her ice chips or juice bars.
- Wipe her face with cool, wet cloths when she is perspiring.
- Let her know if you need to leave the room. Try not to leave her alone during contractions unless she requests it.
- Remind her to pee every hour or so. She may feel only the pressure of the contractions and not realize that her bladder is full.
- Bring her a blanket and socks if she needs them.

To be with the person you love most as she gives birth to your child is a gift and an honor. It can also be a great source of stress. The most difficult part of a partner's role is feeling helpless. There will be times in the labor when you may wish to take away her pain or her work. Know that this is normal.

Be sure to keep your own energy level up by snacking every few hours. Bring food with you from home.

Massage. Massage is a great help in labor. It signals your partner to release muscle tension, it improves her circulation, and it relieves stiffness and discomfort. Before labor begins, practice on each other and talk about what feels best.

Here are a few tips on massaging a woman in labor:

- Work with whatever position she finds most comfortable.
- Use long, flowing strokes. Stroke from the center of her body downward and outward. For example, to massage her arm, start with her shoulder and slowly move down to her elbow, wrist, and fingers.
- Stroke slowly—fewer than ten times per minute—to decrease muscle activity rather than stimulate it.
- Always keep one hand in contact with her skin.
- Use talcum powder or oil to reduce friction.
- Keep your touch light enough to relieve tension, but firm enough to avoid tickling. Very light touch can feel to a woman in active labor a bit like a mosquito buzzing in her ear.
- Use less motion and firmer pressure on her lower back.
- If she is experiencing back labor (page 273), she will probably want firm massage in the lowest part of her back, near her coccyx. Ask her to place your hand on the spot that has the most pressure.

The Panic Routine. Imagine that you and your partner have faithfully attended your childbirth-preparation classes and practiced the relaxation and breathing techniques. Now both of you are at the hospital, and for the past several hours, you have been helping her to cope with labor. Suddenly a contraction overwhelms her. Her breathing changes. It gets noisier and out of rhythm. She may cry out, tense up, or move in an agitated way in the middle of the contraction. When the contraction ends, she says she doesn't think she can handle any more. She is beginning to panic, and you are close to doing the same. What do you do?

Do not wait for full-fledged panic to set in! Your partner is asking for help. She needs more than a pat on the arm. She needs a warm, supportive person to help her regain control. Try this routine:

1. Stand up in front of her. This action says, "I am in charge, and I am going to help you."
2. Get her attention. Say her name, and have her look at you. Bring your face to within 10 inches of hers so that she is looking directly at you.
3. Hold her wrist firmly but gently. This says, "I am here with you."
4. If she is breathing fast or unevenly, breathe with her, and gradually slow your breathing. She will do the same.
5. Talk to her! Praise her efforts with each contraction. If she says, "I didn't handle that contraction very well," tell her that she did just fine. Remind her that the contraction is gone forever, and

Tori's Tip:
Be Good to Yourself

Every night before bed, Alexander and I carry on a tradition that Ray and I started: We lie in the dark and talk about our day. We tell each other three things that happened—the "not-so-best" thing (we get that out of the way first), the funniest thing, and the best thing. This might be your first entry in the journal or scrapbook you keep for your baby. "On the day you were born...

- "the not-so-best thing that happened was...
- "the funniest thing that happened was...
- "the best thing that happened was..."

It might be the start of a nice tradition.

that she'll handle the next one fine. Say that each contraction brings the baby closer. Telling her that you love her may mean more than you could ever imagine.

Treat Her Well. Don't wait until labor to give your sweetie a massage. You might even find for her a massage therapist who specializes in prenatal massage. Your health club may have such a person on staff, or one of her friends may be able to suggest someone.

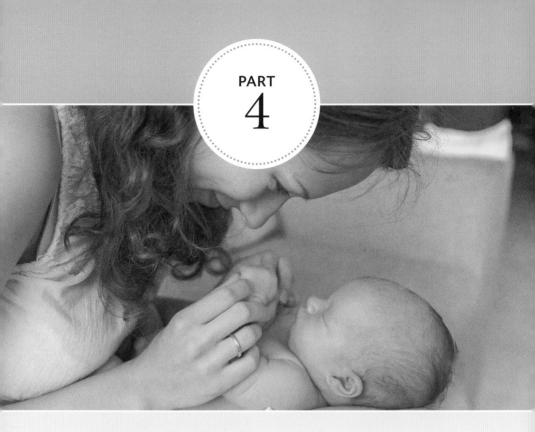

THE FOURTH TRIMESTER

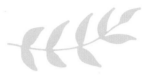

Welcome to Motherhood
THE FIRST MONTH AFTER BIRTH

CONGRATULATIONS! That little being who affected your body so profoundly over the last nine months has finally arrived. His life is just beginning, and yours has changed wonderfully and forever. While you are adjusting to the joy, and shock, of being a new parent, your baby is dealing with the biggest shock of his life—the beginning of life. Learning to live in the world outside your womb is activating all his tender senses. Hearing, smelling, touching, tasting, even watching your face are all astonishing to him.

WHAT'S HAPPENING WITH YOUR BABY?

Babies are generally very alert for the first hour or so after birth. This allows them to adapt to their new surroundings and to have their first feeding at the breast. This is a wonderful time for parents and baby to get to know one another. For help in getting started with breastfeeding, see page 345.

After your milk comes in, your baby will probably urinate eight times a day or more. Less frequent urination could indicate a need for more fluid. Be sure you are feeding your baby at least eight times per day.

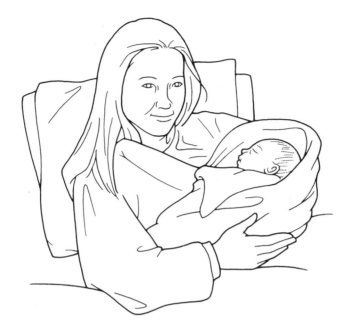

Your baby's first stools will be dark green and tarry meconium (page 158). Over the first week, they will gradually change. If you are breast-feeding, the stools will become yellow and seedy-looking. Initially, your baby should have at least one bowel movement per day, although after the first month, he may poop less often. Some babies poop with every feeding, others once a day, and some just once a week.

Most babies lose a few ounces in the first few days after birth. This is quite normal.

Your baby's umbilical cord should stay dry. Fold the diapers down in front to keep it from getting wet. If you notice bleeding, pus, a foul smell, or a red area on the skin around the base of the cord, call your baby's doctor. The cord will dry up, turn dark brown, and fall off about seven to ten days after birth.

If this is your first baby, getting through the first month will be a considerable accomplishment. There is so much to learn. Here is this brand-new person, your dear little baby, who is, in some ways, like an alien from another planet. You don't speak the same language. You don't eat the same foods. You have many years of experience; to him the world is a complete unknown. Sharing your love and meeting his needs will build a lifetime of caring and trust between you.

Hospital Routines

Your baby will have several tests and other procedures done before going home. Most hospitals and birth centers today encourage moms and babies to remain together during their stay, so most of these procedures will probably be done right at your bedside.

- *An Apgar assessment* of a baby's well-being is done at 1 minute and again at 5 minutes after birth. This very brief assessment helps determine whether the baby needs any immediate medical care. The baby scores 0 to 2 points for each of the following: heart rate, respiratory effort, muscle tone, reflex response, and color. At 5 minutes, most babies score 7, 8, or 9, but few babies score a perfect 10. The Apgar score does not predict a baby's long-term health, intellectual abilities, or behavior.

- *Erythromycin ointment* is placed in the baby's eyes within one to two hours of birth. This is mandated by state laws to prevent bacterial eye infections that could be transmitted from the mother during birth. The ointment does not sting or hurt the baby's eyes, but it will make her vision blurry for a few minutes.

- *Vitamin K injection* isn't mandated by law, but hospitals routinely give babies an injection of vitamin K shortly after birth. This vitamin is an important factor in blood clotting. All babies are deficient in vitamin K, as the body does not manufacture it until several days after birth.

- *Hepatitis B vaccine* is given in the hospital as the first in a series of three vaccines recommended by the American Academy of Pediatrics. Hepatitis B is a serious disease that infects and damages the liver. Transmitted by contact with infected blood or body fluids, the disease is on the increase in the United States. Many states now include the hepatitis B vaccine on the list of immunizations a child must receive before entering kindergarten.

- *Blood tests for congenital disorders* are performed before a baby is discharged from the hospital or birth center. Your baby will receive a small prick on the bottom of her foot (the nurse should first warm your baby's foot to ease the extraction of blood). The blood sample is tested for certain rare diseases. These include *PKU* (*phenylketonuria*), an inability to digest high-protein foods; *hypothyroidism*, low production of thyroid hormone; *galactosemia*, an inability to use some of the sugars in breast milk or formula; and a variety of blood disorders, such as sickle-cell anemia. If left untreated, these disorders can cause mental retardation, seizures, severe illness, or lifelong disabilities. With early testing, many of the disorders can be treated with diet or medications. The baby's doctor will be notified of the test results.

Your Baby's Behavior

From day one, your baby will start to show preferences for things he likes to see, hear, touch, and smell, turning his head toward sounds, changes in light, and new smells. He shows that he recognizes your voice and others' voices that he often heard while in the womb. His body will wriggle, tense up, or visibly relax depending on how he is touched. He is able to see clearly objects approximately 12 to 18 inches (30 to 46 cm) away. That's about the distance from your baby to your face when you are cradling him in your arms. He especially likes to look at sharp contrasts, light and shadow, black and white and red. Most stimulating to a baby's eyes are black and red shapes on a white background. (Alexander loved watching a black and red mobile above his crib. We kept it up until he was old enough to try to pull it down!)

Your newborn has an immense task to carry out—learning to adapt, physically and psychologically, to the mysterious, complex new world into which he has been born. He craves food, comfort, and rest, and he instinctively seeks the bond of love and care with his mother. He will communicate by crying, by tensing his body, by turning his head to track a sound or the nearby scent of his mother's breast. Particularly alert babies may already show signs of mimicry and, sometimes within a few days of birth, will return a smile. Some people say this is the result of intestinal gas, rather than an intentional response, but it sure is a treat for Mom or Dad.

How a baby reacts to his world depends on his personality. During the first month of life, a baby will already manifest certain personality traits. Some new babies are quiet and seem very relaxed; they cry only when they are hungry or uncomfortable. Some are very active, tensing their bodies at the slightest provocation, flailing with their arms and legs, kicking randomly. Still others seem to be in control of their movement from the get-go. There seems to be a deliberation in the way they grip a finger, turn their heads, and react to stimuli in the world around them. They kick regularly and rhythmically, as if moving to some pleasant internal rhythm. Perhaps they have already learned to calm themselves by sucking a thumb or finger.

Each baby is unique. As you learn to read your own baby's body language, you will begin to adjust to his physical needs and create for him the routines that will help him attain optimum well-being and balance, physically and emotionally. For instance, how much does he like to be cuddled, and how does he like to be touched? Some babies like a wide variety of touches, from brisk to gentle; others respond best to one or two types of touching. Your baby's body language will tell you which kind he prefers. Play with him. Play with his fingers and his toes, and blow air gently on his naked skin. Very gentle massage, in a warm, dry room, is a calming, loving way to get him ready for sleep. This is particularly effective with fussy babies. Sing to him; talk to him in a soft voice.

Because each baby is an individual, discovering what your particular baby likes is an adventure for both of you. Walk around the room with him on your shoulder. Cradle him in your arms, and rock him gently back and forth. Sit on your bed with your knees up and support your baby on your thighs as you gently play with his arms and legs and talk to him. Rock with him in a rocking chair, experimenting with different rhythms. Take your baby for a ride in the car. Swing with him in a hammock. Carry your newborn about in a sling and then in a front pack, and see which type of carrier he prefers.

Your Baby's Appearance

You may wonder if some aspects of your baby's appearance are normal. Most likely they are. Here is a list of conditions that are commonly visible in newborns:

Vernix. This thick, creamy white substance protects the baby's skin in the womb. When a baby is born at 40 weeks, vernix is usually seen only in skin folds and creases. But if your baby is born a week or two before your due date, you may notice quite a bit more vernix. Don't try to wash it off. Instead, gently rub it into the baby's skin. It is a wonderful natural lotion.

Bluish hands and feet. As the baby adjusts to circulating her own blood, with no help from the placenta, her hands and feet may appear bluish. This doesn't mean she is cold. The bluish color will go away in a day or two.

Head molding or hematoma. At birth, some babies' heads have a large, round bump (*caput*) or look misshapen because of passage through the pelvic bones. The head will gradually regain its normal shape, often in the first week. If your baby was born with the help of either forceps or a vacuum extractor, she may have superficial marks on the top or sides of her head and face. These will also go away within the first week.

Facial swelling. This is caused by pressure during birth. It subsides within a few days.

Milia. These are small whiteheads on the chin, nose, cheeks, and forehead. When your baby's skin is first exposed to air, her sebaceous (oil) glands may overreact. The pimples will disappear in several days or weeks.

Sucking blister. This is usually caused by the baby's sucking on her upper lip while in the womb.

Peeling skin. Because of the new exposure to air, some babies have dry, peeling skin in the first week of life. You may even notice small cracks in the skin. Ignore these things; they will go away. Babies do not need lotion. Their bodies adjust.

Newborn rash. You may see small, isolated areas of redness, varying in size, on your baby's skin. Tiny bumps may be visible. Spots of rash are usually transient, although new ones may appear for up to ten days.

Breast buds and swollen genitalia. Because of the transfer of maternal hormones, breasts and genitalia may be enlarged in both male and female babies. In girls, these hormones may also cause a slight, pinkish vaginal discharge.

Eye movements. Among newborns, random and jerky movements of the eyes are normal.

Stork bites. These are pale pink or mauve patches that may appear on eyelids or on the back of the neck, especially in light-skinned babies. The patches sometimes fade as the child gets older.

Mongolian spot. This is a purplish brown pigment in the skin of the lower back. These spots are most frequently seen in dark-skinned children.

Lanugo. This fine, downy hair, sometimes barely visible, appears over the shoulders, back, forehead, and cheeks. It is more noticeable in dark-haired babies. Parents are often a bit unnerved to see a beautiful little girl with a furry back! But lanugo rubs off within a couple of days of birth.

Fingernails. In newborns, the nails are paper-thin and often attached to the skin of the fingers. Be careful if you clip them; see page 365 for advice.

Sneezing. Babies sneeze to clear mucus from the nose in the first few days. This is a good sign that all is well.

Jaundice. On the third or fourth day of life, your infant's skin may look yellowish. Your baby's liver may be a little slow in eliminating broken-down red blood cells. Bilirubin, a by-product of broken-down red blood cells, causes the skin to yellow. If you see any change in the color of your baby's skin, let the baby's doctor know. The doctor may want to give the baby a blood test to check her bilirubin level. Frequent feeding reduces jaundice. So does exposure to sunlight; the doctor may have you place the baby by a sunny window for brief periods. If the bilirubin level is quite high, your baby will lie under special lights that help break down bilirubin.

Your Baby's Reflexes

Your baby is born with several neurological reflexes that are part of his brain development. Some are vital to his survival.

Sucking reflex. This reflex is very strong at birth. Any stimulation of a baby's lips elicits sucking motions. Newborns often suck on their thumbs, fingers, or fists. This is probably a continuation of behavior that started before birth.

Swallowing reflex. This is also present prior to birth. In the womb, babies swallow amniotic fluid.

Rooting reflex. If you stroke your baby's cheek, he will turn his head in that direction. To help your baby get started nursing, simply allow your breast to touch his cheek.

Grasp reflex. When you place a finger in your baby's palm, he will grasp your finger tightly. His grasp may be strong enough to allow you to raise his body slightly.

Stepping reflex. If you hold your baby under his arms in a standing position, he will make walking motions.

Moro or startle reflex. If the baby's head is unsupported or his bed is bumped, he will thrust out his arms as if to embrace.

Babinski reflex. If you stroke the sole of your baby's foot, his toes will spread open and the foot will turn slightly inward.

Fencing reflex. This reflex is my favorite. When your baby is on his back and his head turns to one side, he will extend his arm and leg out on that side while the opposite arm and leg bend. He'll look as if he is in a fencing position.

Your Baby's Sleep

Your healthy newborn will spend most of her first month asleep. Newborns sleep an average of 18 hours a day, in 2- to 4-hour stretches. Most babies are alert and eager to interact for only a few minutes at a time. Some babies sleep almost continuously for the first two to three days after birth, awakening only for feedings. If your baby sleeps longer than 3 hours at a stretch, the doctor may recommend waking her for feedings.

Your baby has several sleep-wake states:

- *Drowsiness*, when the baby is falling asleep.

- *Active sleep*, or rapid-eye-movement (REM) sleep. This is typified by irregular breathing and the twitching of muscles. A newborn may cry out in sleep, but this doesn't mean she is uncomfortable or awake. Household noise may awaken her easily during this state, but she will just as easily go back to sleep.

- *Light sleep*, in which the baby is less active and her breathing becomes more regular.

- *Quiet sleep*, or deep sleep. The baby breathes regularly and makes no movement except for occasional, sudden body jerks. Normal household noise will not awaken her during this time.

- *Wide awake.* In this state, the baby quietly watches people and things around her, smiles, and, as she becomes older, explores her hands and feet.

If your baby has trouble falling asleep, you can help her relax. Play soft recorded sounds—soothing music, waves, wind in the trees, or a heartbeat—or place a ticking clock by her bed. By feeding and diapering her quietly at night, with minimal lighting, you help her begin to learn that nighttime and daytime are different.

What should your baby wear for sleeping? If the room temperature is between 68 and 75° F (20 to 24° C), your baby will be comfortable in just a diaper and a shirt or gown, with a light cotton blanket as cover.

Dressing your baby lightly lessens her risk of succumbing to Sudden Infant Death Syndrome (SIDS; see page 41). There are several other steps you can take to decrease this risk: Lay her on her back for nighttime sleep and naps, without any pillows under or around her.

Throughout the day, have your baby on her side and belly to be sure she is frequently in different positions. Keep any lambskin, stuffed animals, or fluffy blankets out of her bed, and avoid overheating the room. Keep secondhand smoke out of the house. Breastfeeding may also lessen your baby's risk of SIDS.

Your Baby's Crying

Crying is your baby's primary tool for communicating with you. Babies cry for many reasons—hunger, discomfort from wetness, a bowel movement, gas, fatigue. Figuring out why your baby is crying will be one of the greatest challenges of the first month. There are no sure-fire techniques for soothing an uncomfortable baby. Often you must try one thing and, if it doesn't work, try another, in a process of elimination. Soon you will be able to interpret your baby's cries easily, most of the time.

If your baby is colicky, he'll cry a lot. Most people define *colic* as crying that continues for several hours without stop each day, often at the same time of day; doesn't respond to the usual comfort measures; and usually lessens after about three months of age. Many think the cause is abdominal cramps, but no one knows what causes the cramps. Colic has been linked to the endocrine system, the digestive system, the mother's hormones, and the immaturity of the baby's intestines. Some babies seem to have more trouble than others do in adjusting to the digestive process.

If your breastfed baby occasionally gets fussy and you can't figure out why, try to remember what you ate an hour or two before a fussy period began. Foods that often irritate babies include dairy products, tomatoes, citrus, cabbage, broccoli, garlic, onions, beans, and chocolate. If you suspect one of these foods or something else in your diet, see if your baby reacts when you eat the suspect food again.

Fussy bottle-fed babies may benefit from switching formulas. It's best to consult the baby's doctor, however, before choosing a new product.

Because the cause of colic is still not well understood, the only proven treatment for a colicky baby is a "tincture of time." Meanwhile, you can develop a bag of tricks to cope with the crying until your baby matures; see the list on page 334 for ideas.

Tori's Tip:
Ways to Soothe a Crying Baby

- Unless you've fed the baby recently, always try feeding first.
- Check the baby's diaper. Wet diapers bother some babies, although most infants don't mind. Babies often poop while being fed; you can tell this is happening by the red face, the grunting, or both (this is a reason to feed the baby before the diaper change).
- Offer the breast or formula again after the diaper change.
- Burp the baby halfway through the feeding and again at the end.
- Cuddle the baby while you're sitting or lying down.
- Try swaddling (page 360). This makes a baby feel as if she's still in your womb.
- Movement frequently does the trick. Rock or gently bounce the baby, or let her sway in an infant swing. Slip her into a sling or front pack or stroller, and go for a walk. If you're really desperate, put her into her car seat and go for a drive.
- Encourage your baby to suck on her fingers, your (clean) finger, or a pacifier.

WHAT'S HAPPENING WITH YOUR BODY?

Your body will go through many changes once the baby is born. The following pages tell you what to expect and discuss how to take care of yourself during this time of adjustment.

Your Breasts

Initially, your breasts will produce *colostrum*, the first and perfect food for your baby. Because this yellowish, thick, high-protein fluid is concentrated, it is produced in small quantities.

- Hold your baby close with her ear to your chest, so she can hear your heartbeat.
- Remove unnecessary stimuli. Dim the lights, turn off the television, and keep visitors to a minimum.
- Gently massage the baby's abdomen, or lay her across your knees, tummy-side down, and rub her back.
- Sing her a lullaby, or play soft music.
- Try white noise, such as the distant sound of a hair dryer, washing machine, or vacuum cleaner. If your baby likes it—and you'd be surprised at how many do—record the sound so that you can play it continuously without wearing out your appliances!

If all these strategies fail, your baby may simply be overtired. Put her down in a crib or bassinet. After a few minutes of fussing, she may just conk out on her own.

For a baby with colic or inconsolable crying that intensifies or persists throughout the day, you'll want to consult your baby's doctor to rule out any medical problem.

Your mature milk will "come in" approximately 48 to 72 hours after birth. When this happens, your breasts may become *engorged*—swollen, very firm, and a little sore. Frequent nursing will help keep your breasts soft. Engorgement can occur quite suddenly; to keep it from worsening, you may wish to wake your baby to nurse. You should certainly offer the breast each time your baby wakes or seems hungry. (For more about breastfeeding, see page 345.) Warm washcloths placed on your breasts will keep your milk flowing freely and help prevent *mastitis*, or breast infection. Mastitis manifests itself as a tender, reddened area of the breast, along with fever, headache, and other flulike symptoms.

Your body will initiate milk production even if you have decided against breastfeeding. In this case, you will want to wear a snug-fitting bra to minimize engorgement and discomfort. Applying ice packs will also help decrease the swelling.

Your Uterus

During late pregnancy, your uterus is about the size of a basketball. Right after birth, it should shrink to the size of a grapefruit and sit just below your navel. Then it will gradually returns to its pre-pregnant size, approximately that of a small pear.

If your uterus doesn't contract enough to become very firm when your baby is born, you could have excessive bleeding from the site where the placenta was attached. In this case, your nurse or other practitioner will press on your abdomen above your navel until the uterus becomes firm. He or she will have you feel for the "grapefruit" and show you how to massage it yourself. It is important that your uterus remain firm in the few days after birth.

Breastfeeding releases oxytocin, which causes the uterus to continue contracting. Pitocin (page 311), that is, synthetic oxytocin, is frequently given immediately after birth to ensure that the uterus remains firm.

Within a couple of hours after birth, you may experience uncomfortable contractions that feel like menstrual cramps, often referred to as *afterpains*. These may be more noticeable when you nurse your baby, because of the natural release of oxytocin. Applying a warm heating pack or pad to your abdomen can help relieve this discomfort. You can also take 600 milligrams of ibuprofen every 4 to 6 hours, as recommended by your practitioner, to decrease the cramping.

Bleeding

The vaginal discharge after birth is called *lochia*. This is a combination of the uterine lining and blood. Your lochia will probably change from bright red to pink to whitish over the course of several weeks. Initially it will be quite heavy, much like the heaviest day of your menstrual period. If your bleeding subsides and then increases again, decrease your activity; this is your body's way of telling you to slow down and rest more. Use sanitary pads instead of tampons until your bleeding has completely subsided. Vaginal bleeding after a cesarean birth will usually be less than after a vaginal birth.

Perineal Tear

If you have had a perineal tear or an episiotomy, your practitioner may have placed several stitches in your perineum. A very small vaginal tear may not require any stitches. After you urinate, you should rinse with a wet cloth or a squirt bottle of water, or pat the area with a witch hazel-soaked pad (such as Tucks), to relieve any stinging. For the first day or two, you may also wish to use an ice pack for comfort and to decrease swelling. After that, you might use a portable sitz bath (a tub for sitting in) or sit in warm, shallow water in a bathtub. This will not only provide comfort but also help promote healing by bringing extra blood flow to the area. Your stitches do not need to be removed; they will dissolve in about two weeks. Your perineum should heal very well within about two to three weeks.

Hemorrhoids

Hemorrhoids are varicose veins of the rectum. Some women develop hemorrhoids during pregnancy or while giving birth, because of the weight and pressure of the baby and the force of pushing. Hemorrhoid pain may be relieved with ice packs, witch hazel, or a cream prescribed by your practitioner. Try to avoid becoming constipated, as this can aggravate the discomfort or cause the hemorrhoids to bleed. Hemorrhoids will eventually shrink and become less uncomfortable.

Taking Care of Yourself

Do you feel as if you've just run the Boston Marathon on two hours of sleep? You've done one of the most challenging things a human being can do. Your baby will be happiest if you take good care of yourself now.

Rest is crucial. Sleep when the baby sleeps. This is easier said than done, of course. I was running around with Alexander two weeks after we came home from the hospital. When he was three weeks old, I developed a bladder infection for the first time and mastitis. I quickly realized how much healing I needed to do. My body was crying out for rest. After that, Alexander and I had a nap schedule.

It's wonderful if you have a partner who can stay home or close family or friends who can take care of you for a while, but not all of us do. Now is the time to keep a phone-side list of local restaurants that deliver. Now is also the time to call in the favors of any people who told you that they'd be glad to help when the baby arrived. Help can come in many forms and can make a big difference in easing you through

Tori's Tip:
Avoid Constipation

Your bowels probably emptied themselves before or during labor, so don't be surprised if you have no bowel movement for the first day or two after birth. It is important, however, to avoid becoming constipated. Here are some things that will help:

- Try not to let fear of pain or discomfort keep you from having a bowel movement. Holding in a bowel movement can increase the likelihood of becoming constipated.
- Eat high-fiber foods such as fresh fruits, vegetables, and whole grains.
- Drink plenty of fluids.
- Walk as much as you comfortably can.
- Add prunes and bran to your diet, if needed, to keep your stools soft.
- Ask your practitioner about taking a stool softener if these methods are not enough.

this transition. My girlfriends and I—we called ourselves the Sanity Sisters—have a special tradition for when a friend has a baby. Each day during the first week that the baby is home, one of us will prepare an entire dinner for the family, including salad, bread, and dessert. We bring it to the mother's house, give her and the baby a kiss, and leave. The family has nearly a week of wonderful, home-cooked meals. I will never forget that precious week.

Without strong support from family and friends, a hired postpartum doula can be a godsend during the first couple of weeks. Postpartum doulas typically come into your home for a few hours each day and assist with baby care, breastfeeding, and light house hold chores. You can find these postpartum services through your childbirth educator or birth facility.

Especially if you are breastfeeding, eating nutritious foods is still very important. Many women are intimidated by the thought that they must maintain a perfect diet while they are nursing. Try not to worry. Simply include plenty of protein (whether in the form of steak or peanut butter), grains, vegetables, and fruits. If you maintained a well-balanced diet during your pregnancy, you are probably already eating well. It helps to keep on hand a supply of nutritious snacks, such as nuts, hard-boiled eggs, yogurt, and cheese. You will need to consume extra calories, about 500 more per day than before pregnancy, and you should continue to take a prenatal vitamin to meet your body's increased need for vitamins A and B12.

If you are breastfeeding, you will probably find that you are thirstier than usual. Your body needs increased fluid to maintain adequate milk production. An easy way to keep up is to drink a glass of water each time you sit down to nurse your baby.

You may find yourself going through an emotional wringer. As your hormones readjust themselves, you may feel moody for no apparent reason. Trust that these swings are normal and will pass. If, however, you find yourself unable to function, crying excessively each day, or not wishing to care for your baby, you should talk about this with your practitioner.

Hormones are also the reason that you may wake up drenched with perspiration during the first two weeks. Your body is responding to *prolactin*, a breastfeeding hormone, as well as eliminating excess fluid that you retained during your pregnancy.

As you care for your infant, baby yourself as much as possible. Taking a hot bath not only feels good but is also very healing. Have someone watch the baby while you bathe, if possible, or place the baby in an infant seat next to the bath. Taking a bath with the baby is wonderful, but a little time alone in the tub is also very important for you. Remember, caring for yourself and your baby is much more important than keeping the house in order.

IMPORTANT THINGS TO KNOW

So often, new parents wonder how they will learn, recognize, and care for their baby's many needs. Rest assured that even if you have never before cared for an infant, you will very quickly learn what works for your own child.

How to Pick Up and Hold Your Baby

He is tiny. He is vulnerable. But he is not as delicate as he seems. These simple pointers will help you learn to hold your infant with confidence.

To avoid startling a newborn, always lift him slowly. If he is awake, first make your presence known through eye contact or a cheerful greeting. Then ease the transition from mattress to your arms by placing your hands under his back and leaving them there for several moments before you try to lift him. When you're ready to pick him up, lean in as close as possible to reduce the time your baby spends traveling through the air.

Until your baby can hold his head up on his own, you'll need to support it by cradling his neck with your hand or arm. Beyond that, you can experiment until you find a position that your baby likes. Some want to be snuggled close; others are happiest when facing the world. Here are three common holds you can try:

What If You Get to Go Home Before Your Twins Do?

Twins often come early, and sometimes they have to spend a little more time in the hospital than do most full-term babies. Before babies are discharged from the hospital, they must meet several general criteria: They must weigh enough (frequently, over 4 pounds [1.8 kg]), suck adequately, and be able to regulate and maintain their body temperature. If you are discharged from the hospital before your babies are, I urge you to take advantage of this time to catch up on sleep and recover from the birth, because you'll need every ounce of energy when your babies do come home. Some hospitals offer a special room for parents to stay in while their babies are in the neonatal intensive care unit (NICU) or transitional nursery; you may be able to choose between staying here and going home for the night. Either way, if the NICU nurses are willing to cover for you during the night, take them up on it (accept all offers of help!). The babies are in expert hands, and by relying on those hands, you will be well rested and better prepared to handle all those nights at home when you don't have such help.

The cradle hold. Let the baby rest his head in the crook of your arm. Use your free hand to support his bottom and back.

The tummy hold. Balance your baby face down on one arm, using the crook of your arm to support his neck. His chest and abdomen should rest on your forearm. For additional support, place your free hand between your baby's legs and under your other arm. This position, sometimes called the colic hold, can be particularly soothing to a baby with a gassy tummy.

The shoulder hold. Use one hand to support your baby's neck while holding it against your shoulder. Use your free hand to support your baby's bottom.

When you lay your newborn back down again, keep your hands underneath him for a few moments. This will make the transition from arms back to mattress less disturbing.

Circumcision

The removal of the foreskin—the sheath of tissue covering the head of the penis—has been known since ancient times, when it was performed as a religious rite or as an initiation of boys into adulthood. Many parents today still have their sons circumcised, for religious or other reasons. In the United States, the practice is less popular today than it was 50 years ago, when it was nearly universal, but in some regions of the country, circumcision is still very popular. Most U.S. circumcisions are performed in the hospital one or two days after birth.

Circumcision has some advantages. The procedure prevents infection and inflammation of the foreskin and may prevent other diseases as well. It seems to decrease the risk of cancer of the penis, although this disease is very rare, occurring in fewer than 1 in 100,000 men in the United States. Some studies have shown a greater risk of cervical cancer in women whose male partners are infected with genital human papilloma virus (HPV) when those partners are uncircumcised. Circumcision may reduce a man's risk of contracting and passing on sexually transmitted diseases. Safe sexual practices, however, are far more important than circumcision in preventing transmission of these diseases, and a new vaccine can provide women partial protection from HPV.

Occasionally, problems with the uncircumcised penis can require circumcision at an older age. These problems, which include recurrent episodes of infection or inflammation of the foreskin or adherence of the foreskin to the tip of the penis, occur in 2 to 6 percent of uncircumcised males.

Like any minor surgery, circumcision poses some risk of complications. Excessive bleeding or infection occurs in fewer than 1 in 1,000 cases.

As you might expect, circumcision is painful. To reduce pain during the procedure, local anesthesia is frequently used. If you want to have your son circumcised, you might talk with your baby's doctor about whether anesthesia will be used.

After your son's circumcision, the edge of his penis will be red. The penis will also be swollen for about 24 hours, and you may notice some oozing. During diaper changes, apply petroleum jelly to the penis to prevent irritation and to keep the diaper from sticking. As the penis heals, a soft, yellowish crust will form. Gently clean the penis with warm water. If at any time, bleeding begins and will not stop with gentle pressure, call your baby's doctor.

If you do not have your son circumcised, you will not need to do anything to his penis except to keep it clean. Wash the outside with soap and water during his bath. Never forcibly retract the foreskin, which is usually joined to the glans during infancy. The foreskin will loosen by itself, probably by the time your son is three or four years old.

Since there are no strong medical reasons to circumcise or not, your decision regarding circumcision is a personal one. Make the choice with which you are most comfortable.

Tori's Tip:
Know When to Call the Baby's Doctor

It is very important to get in touch with your doctor if your baby shows any of the following:

- Excessive and prolonged crying or unusual irritability
- Excessive drowsiness (sleeping during times that the baby is usually awake)
- Frequent waking and general restlessness
- Refusal to nurse, or significant or sudden loss of appetite
- Significant decline in urination (fewer than five wet diapers per day)
- Repeated vomiting
- Fever higher than 101°F (38°C)
- Stools that contain blood, mucus, or pus or are liquid, foul smelling, or continuous
- Coughing or a prolonged runny nose, especially with malaise
- Redness or swelling in one or both eyes, or discharge from the eye or eyes
- Hoarseness, wheezing, or difficulty breathing
- Rash, especially if it is over a large portion of the body (beware of possible allergies to laundry detergents or lotions)
- Convulsions, unusual twitching, or an inability to move
- Apparent pain, of any kind, that is not resolved with tender loving care

Always check with your pediatrician before giving your newborn any medication.

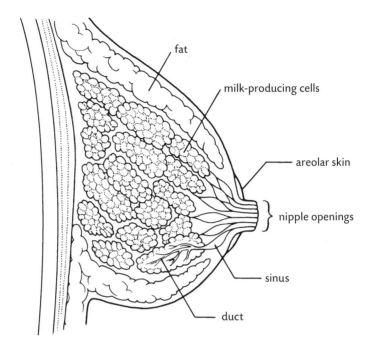

fat

milk-producing cells

areolar skin

nipple openings

sinus

duct

Breastfeeding Basics

On page 209, I described the benefits your baby receives from breast-feeding. There are also benefits for *you*. You can breastfeed anywhere, anytime. There is no formula to mix or bottles to clean. The extra 500 calories of food you'll need each day are far less expensive than baby formula. And nursing time is a pleasurable, close time between you and your baby.

MILK PRODUCTION IN YOUR BREASTS

The breast is perfectly designed for feeding. The tiny bumps on the *areola*—the dark or pinkish circle around the nipple—secrete a lubricant that keeps the tissue soft and bacteria-free. Milk production works as a supply-and-demand system; the more you feed your baby, the more milk you will make. Breast size has nothing to do with how much milk your body can produce.

YOUR MILK

The first milk your body produces, colostrum, is a thick, yellowish fluid with the perfect combination of nutrients for your baby's first several days of life. Although colostrum is produced in small amounts to suit your baby's small stomach, this first food is high in protein and easily digestible. It also contains antibodies, which help protect the baby from infection.

Tori's Tip:
Learn to Take the Baby's Temperature

If you suspect that your baby is ill, take her temperature before calling your baby's doctor. You will want to keep a digital thermometer handy. Follow the directions that come with it.

For an axillary (underarm) temperature, place the thermometer under one of the baby's arms, with the tip in the armpit. An axillary temperature is usually a little lower than a rectal temperature.

If you have never taken a rectal temperature, your baby's doctor can show you how.

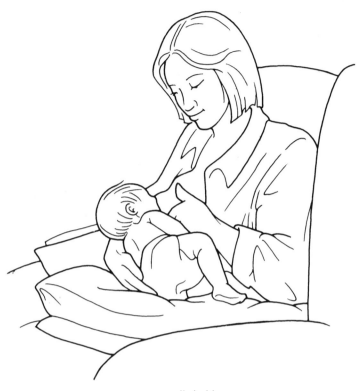

cradle hold

After the first few days, your body makes mature milk. Each time you nurse your baby, the milk starts out thin and bluish. This *foremilk*, which contains lactose and proteins but very little fat, satisfies the baby's initial hunger and thirst. When the baby is nearly done with the feeding, the milk he withdraws is called the *hind milk*. This milk contains more fat, which is your baby's main source of energy. It keeps your baby satisfied until the next feeding.

HOLDING THE BABY FOR FEEDING

You can use several different positions for breastfeeding:

With the *cradle hold*, you hold your baby in the crook of your arm, with her head at your elbow and her belly against yours.

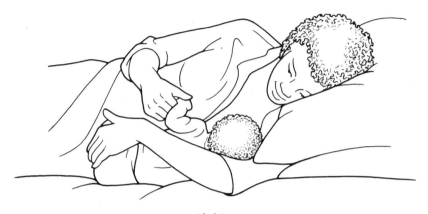

side lying

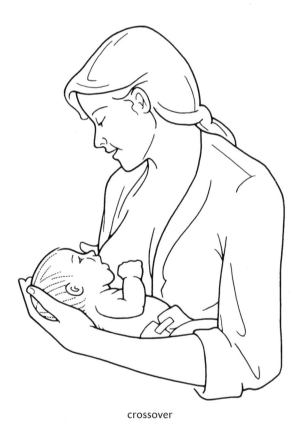

crossover

Side lying is a comfortable position, especially for nighttime feedings or after a cesarean.

With the *crossover* or *cross-cradle hold,* you again support your baby with your arm, but this time, her feet are at your elbow and your hand supports her head. Especially with a small baby or one who has difficulty latching on this hold makes it easy to guide her mouth to the breast on the side of your body opposite your supporting arm.

With the *football hold,* you tuck the baby under your arm like a football, with her head resting on your hand and facing up and her body supported by your forearm. This position is excellent if you're recovering from a cesarean section, because it keeps the weight of the baby off your tender abdomen.

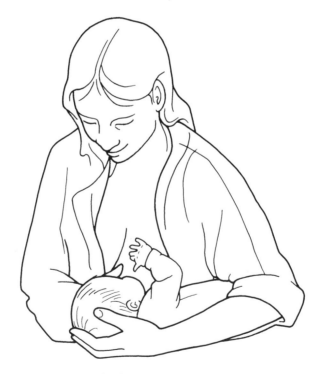

football hold

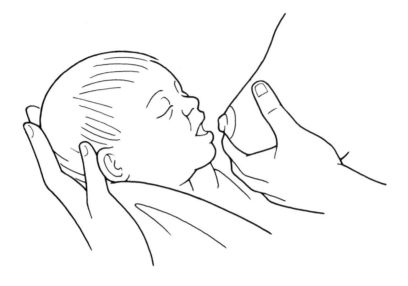

POSITIONING THE BABY AT THE BREAST

Hold the baby close, with his chest and nose touching your breast. With one hand, support the baby's neck and head; with the other, gently lift your breast. Touch your nipple to your baby's cheek in an upward motion, until he opens his mouth wide. Bring him onto your breast, placing as much of the areola in his mouth as possible. If your breast is very full, you may need to compress it, with your fingers at the edge of the areola. This makes it easier for the baby to latch on. Positioning the baby correctly at the breast is the single most important way to prevent soreness of the nipples.

Yes, You Can Breastfeed Both Your Babies!

Breastfeeding twins is a special experience. Some women find it to be very challenging, but others find it to be the easiest way to feed their babies. If you are pregnant with twins, I strongly suggest taking a breastfeeding class and speaking directly with a lactation specialist. She can show you how to latch two babies on at the same time. The consultant can help you with proper pumping techniques, if you wish to use bottles. Pumping your milk will allow your spouse and family members to feed the babies, and take a lot of pressure off you. To breastfeed your twins, it's good to have the following items on hand:

- A breastfeeding pillow designed for twins
- A high-quality electric double breast pump for fast and efficient pumping
- A bottle-propping pillow, to hold a bottle for one baby when you are feeding the other one

When your baby is latched on correctly, both his lips will pout, and he will make quiet swallowing sounds. If you hear smacking noises, he is not latched on properly; take him off and try again. Your baby's nose is designed so that he will usually have no trouble breathing, but if it seems compressed against your breast, you can gently press down against the breast to give the nose more room.

LETDOWN REFLEX

Shortly after your baby latches on and begins sucking, you may feel a tingle in your breast. This is your milk "letting down." Your baby will start swallowing rapidly, and milk may leak or spray from the free breast.

Sometimes your milk may let down when you hear your baby cry or when a longer time than usual has passed between feedings. It is helpful to wear nursing pads—either disposable or washable cloth ones—to absorb the milk that may drip from your breasts at these times as well as during feedings.

SORE NIPPLES

Nipple soreness occurs primarily when the baby latches on during the first few days of breastfeeding. If the baby is positioned correctly on the breast, the soreness may last only a few seconds. If the baby is positioned incorrectly, the soreness will continue, and the nipple may crack and bleed.

Prevention is the best way to manage soreness. Be certain that the baby latches on to your breast properly. The baby's lips should pull on your areola, not on your nipple. Your nipple should be far back in the baby's mouth during each feeding.

Here are ways to help prevent and minimize nipple soreness:

- Use only clear water to wash your breasts. Do not use soap or lotion on them.
- Whenever possible, allow your nipples to air-dry after feedings.
- Change nursing pads often to keep your breasts as dry as possible.
- Begin each feeding on the least sore side.
- If the baby doesn't release the nipple on her own, break the suction with your finger before removing the baby from the breast.
- Put a warm compress on the sore breast just before each feeding.
- If your nipples are cracked or bleeding, rub a small amount of purified, medical-grade lanolin on them after each feeding. Modified lanolin is available in many drugstores and on the Internet.
- Acetaminophen or ibuprofen can be helpful for pain.

Formula-Feeding Basics

Breast milk is ideally suited for your infant's nutritional needs; it is the food nature intends for babies. Manufactured formulas, however, can also meet your baby's nutritional needs. Your baby's doctor can guide you in choosing the appropriate formula for your infant.

There are two common types of formulas. Milk-based formulas are standard. They are made from heat-treated cow's milk, to which vegetable oils, vitamins, and minerals are added. Soy-based formulas are recommended for babies who can't tolerate cow's milk. Soy formulas contain higher levels of protein than standard milk-based formulas contain, because soy protein is not as easily absorbed as milk protein. In addition to these two common types, special formulas are available for premature infants and for those with metabolic disorders.

Milk-based formulas come with or without added iron. The American Academy of Pediatrics recommends iron-fortified formula for all infants who are formula fed.

Formulas come in ready-to-feed, liquid concentrate, and powdered forms. Be sure to follow the manufacturer's recommendations and instructions for preparing each kind. Here are some general rules to follow:

- Wash and rinse the bottles, nipples, mixing utensils, and measuring cups in warm, soapy water, or run them through a complete dishwasher cycle (rubber nipples should be washed by hand). Be sure no milk residue remains on the nipples or necks of the bottles. A bottle brush will come in handy. Ask your baby's doctor whether it is necessary for you to sterilize bottles or nipples.
- Boil water for 5 minutes, and then let it cool before combining it with formula powder or concentrate. Boiled water can be stored in the refrigerator, covered, for up to two days.
- Always refrigerate formula after preparing it, and be sure to use it within 48 hours.
- Never heat your baby's bottle in the microwave oven. Because microwaves heat unevenly, they can cause glass bottles to explode and plastic ones to melt.
- If your baby does not finish the entire bottle, throw the rest away, since bacteria can grow in the bottle.

Notify your baby's doctor if your baby shows any possible signs of formula intolerance or allergy, such as excessive spitting up, vomiting, diarrhea, or skin reactions.

Burping Your Baby

When drinking breast milk or formula, your baby will swallow some air. Some babies swallow much more air than others do. When air bubbles form in your baby's tummy, she is bound to start fussing. Fortunately, you can help her pass that air if you learn how and when to burp her. If your baby is breastfed, burp her before switching breasts and at the end of each feeding. If you are bottle-feeding, stop for a burping break halfway through the feeding time; for example, if your baby drinks 2 ounces (59 ml), burp her after 1 ounce (29 ml). If you see any sign of discomfort, stop sooner.

One reason that babies suck is to comfort themselves, and some infants desire more frequent sucking than others. One baby may use his thumb or hand, while another may not. If your baby doesn't easily soothe himself, introducing a pacifier is perfectly sensible. But introduce a pacifier only after breastfeeding is well established, generally no earlier than two to three weeks after birth. Don't wait too long, however; after four to six weeks of breastfeeding, many babies will not accept an artificial nipple.

There are three good positions for burping a baby. Try them all, and decide which works best for you.

The shoulder burp. Rest your infant's head against your shoulder, using your hand and forearm to support her bottom. Be sure that her breathing is not obstructed. With the palm of your free hand, firmly but gently pat her back, or rub her back in an upward motion.

The sitting burp. Hold your baby so that she is sitting upright. Until she has gained control of her neck muscles, you'll need to support her head by holding it slightly forward and cupping her chin between your thumb and forefinger. With your other hand, firmly pat her back.

The lap burp. Lay your infant across your lap, tummy-side down, with her arms extended and her head to the side. Raise one of your legs so that her head and chest are elevated. Use one hand to steady her and the other to firmly pat her back.

If, after several minutes of waiting, you still don't hear a belch, give up. No baby burps at every feeding.

Many babies spit up after feeding. This is normal, but repeated or projectile vomiting should be reported to your baby's doctor.

Diapering Your Baby

Newborns go through 10 to 12 diapers a day, so even if you've never changed a diaper before having your own baby, you'll quickly learn the tricks of the trade. In the meantime, these simple directions can make your early attempts less taxing.

Lay your infant on his back in a safe, flat place. Unless you're using the floor or the ground, keep one hand on your baby at all times.

Unfasten the used diaper. If your baby has had a bowel movement, wipe away most of the feces with the front, unsoiled part of the diaper.

Gently remove the remaining stool with commercial baby wipes or a soft, damp cloth. To thoroughly clean the baby's bottom, lift him up by his ankles. Then clean the baby's genitals and the surrounding skin with a clean wipe. If your baby is a girl, make sure her labia are clean, and be sure to wipe from front to back to prevent bacteria from entering the vagina. With a boy, lay a cloth diaper or washcloth over the penis to prevent an unexpected shower.

To prevent or treat diaper rash, *apply an ointment* such as Aquaphor, A+D ointment, Balmex, or Desitin to his bottom.

Open a fresh diaper, and slide it underneath your baby. If it's a disposable, the tabs go underneath your baby's back. Pull the diaper up between your baby's legs and to his waist. When diapering a boy, first position his penis down into the diaper so that urine won't seep out the top. If your baby's umbilical stump hasn't fallen off yet, turn down the top edge of the diaper to expose the cord to the air. If you're using a disposable diaper, open the adhesive tabs, and fasten each one tightly across the front. Do the same for a cloth diaper, but pin the diaper in place instead of using tape, or else use a diaper cover with Velcro-type fasteners. If you are using safety pins, place your own fingers between your baby's flesh and the diaper when you insert the pin into the diaper. This way, if you slip with the pin, you stab yourself and not the baby.

Check how much space is between the baby's thighs and the diaper. It should fit snugly but not pinch or bind. You should just be able to fit one finger between the diaper and your baby. If the diaper doesn't fit quite right, unfasten it and make the necessary adjustments before refastening.

Tori's Tip:
Don't Leave Home without It!

Your diaper bag, that is, not your American Express card. You and your newborn can easily go on short outings with minimal supplies—a couple of diapers, a change of clothes, and a light blanket. For longer outings—say, a half-day or more—you'll want to pack a bag. I have often said that less is best, and a diaper bag can be heavy to carry around. If you are traveling by car, though, your life will be easier and your outings more pleasant if you are well organized and well stocked. Here is a foolproof guide to stocking your diaper bag. Happy packing!

- *At least three disposable or four cloth diapers.* What you don't wrap around your baby's bottom you may need to clean up spit-up, spills, and random goo.
- *At least two diaper covers,* if you are using cloth diapers.
- *A plastic-coated changing pad,* either attached to the diaper bag or tucked in separately.
- *Two plastic zipper bags.* They are the easiest way to transport soiled diapers without smelling up the entire car.
- *Baby wipes.* These are indispensable.
- *Diaper ointment,* if your baby has a rash.
- *At least two changes of baby clothes.* (When Alexander was six months old, we went out for an afternoon of errands. I had brought one change of clothes for him. Alexander had a diaper leak that took care of the clothes he was wearing. Then he threw up all over the next set. I had to leave those clothes on him until we got home. I felt that everyone who saw us must have been thinking, "How can she keep that baby in such filthy clothes?")
- *An extra sweater,* a receiving blanket, or both.
- *Nursing pads.* The ones you are wearing are likely to get soaked if you are in a checkout line or driving when your milk lets down.

- *A hat with a brim or earflaps*, depending on the time of year. Never mind that your baby will probably pull it off and fling it into the middle of a crowded street as soon as you put it on his head.
- *Baby sun block*, after the first six months, in case you are out in the sun longer than expected. There will be wonderful moments of bonding for you and your baby as you smear it on him in public while he shrieks.
- *Two extra pacifiers,* if your baby uses them. If he does—trust me— you will never want to be without.
- *Formula*, if you are using it. Bring at least two feedings' worth and an ice pack. Some companies make to-go packs of formula that are easily mixed with water, but these are more expensive.
- *One extra empty bottle*, if you are formula feeding. (My friend Julia's baby threw his bottle across the seat and out of the car window. Pretty good shot for an eight-month-old!)
- *The phone number for your baby's doctor.* If you have a cellular phone, key in the number.

For parents of an older baby or a toddler, a diaper bag is a Winnebago with a zipper. When your baby is about six months old, you'll start stuffing in Cheerios, crackers, string cheese, tofu cubes (some kids love them, no fooling), tubs of applesauce or yogurt, a baby spoon. You'll also want at least a couple of compact toys to amuse your baby when boredom sets in. Otherwise, she will play with the contents of your handbag (inspecting the pictures of U.S. presidents in your wallet and then watching them blow away in the wind will particularly amuse her).

In packing your diaper bag, try to be as thorough as a court-appointed accountant. Too many parents have been stuck in a car, a restaurant, or a childless relative's home when the baby is having a meltdown and they discover they have committed the cardinal sin of P.I.S.S.—Packed Insufficient Supplies and Snacks!

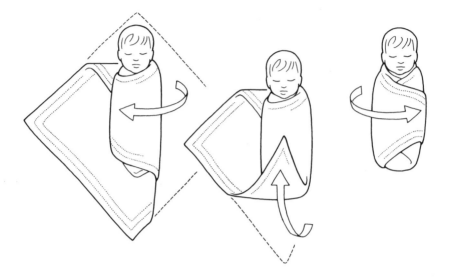

Swaddling Your Baby

Bright lights, loud noises, and endless space. The womb-to-world leap can sometimes be unsettling for a newborn. But snugly wrapping your baby in a soft receiving blanket can simulate the place she once called home.

Here is how to swaddle your baby:

1. Lay a receiving blanket down on a flat surface. Fold down the top left corner. Position the baby on the blanket diagonally, with her head resting just above the folded corner.
2. Wrap her left arm against her left side by pulling the blanket over her torso and tucking the edge of the blanket under her back on her right side.
3. Lift the bottom end of the blanket up towards her midsection so that it covers her feet and tummy.
4. Hold her right arm against her right side as you pull the right side of the blanket snugly across the chest and tuck it around her left side.

Of course, not all babies enjoy a good swaddle. Pay attention to your newborn's signals to find out what suits her.

Dressing and Undressing Your Baby

In the early weeks of parenting, dressing a newborn can seem like a monumental task. It sometimes takes parents a while to feel comfortable maneuvering their baby's tiny hands and limbs through clothes. Your baby may resist stretching out and may react against the cool air on his skin. Some newborns startle easily when moved for dressing. Here are a few tips to make the process easier.

- Choose clothing with quick-change features. Your best bet is stretch suits, with or without legs, with zippers or snaps up the front and in the crotch. The easiest way to get one of these suits on the baby is by laying down the open garment and then placing your infant on top. Use one hand to guide your baby's arm through the sleeve. Use the other hand to reach through the cuff, and gently pull his arm through the opening. (When your baby is older, you can even make a game of this: "Where's Baby's hand? Here it is!") Insert the baby's legs after his arms, if the suit has legs, and then zip or snap up the suit.

- Don't buy garments with stiff seams or tight arms and legs. And, for safety's sake, avoid anything with long ribbons or strings. These can be a choking hazard. A short ribbon, such as on a kimono, is fine as long as it is tied securely.

- At night, it may be very convenient to dress the baby in a gown with elastic or a drawstring at the bottom. This allows for easy diaper changes.

- Shirts that must be drawn over the head can be scary for a baby. It helps if the garment has a generous or expandable neck. In any case, you'll want to stretch the opening as wide as it will go before sliding it over your baby's head. Use your fingers to keep the material from catching on his face.

- For pants, reach into a bottom leg opening, and reach upward to find the baby's foot. Then gently guide his foot down through the opening and insert the other foot the same way before pulling the pants up.

A simple rule for keeping your baby warm is this: He needs one more layer than you do. (Unless you're going to Grandma's, in which case, add three sweaters and a snowsuit!)

Bathing Your Baby

Alexander has always been a little fish; he has loved his baths from his very first one. Most babies come to love their baths, but in the early weeks, some babies complain a bit about this new experience.

Until your newborn's umbilical stump falls off (and his penis heals, if he has had a circumcision), you can keep your little one squeaky-clean with sponge baths. Before you get started, you'll want to ready all your equipment: a hooded towel, a washcloth, baby shampoo and a mild glycerin soap (if you think you need them), a fresh diaper, and a basin or tub of warm water. To make sure the water isn't too hot for the baby's sensitive skin, test it by dipping your elbow or your inner wrist in it. Here are the simple steps to follow for baby's sponge bath:

1. Undress your baby down to her diaper, and wrap her in a warm towel. Lay her on a padded surface such as a changing table. Keep one hand on her at all times.
2. Dip a washcloth in the warm water, and wring it out slightly. Then gently swab your baby's eyes to remove any discharge, always wiping from the inside corner out. Clean the rest of her face, and pat it dry. Next, rub some soap onto the washcloth, if she is sticky with milk, and clean her neck, chest, back, arms, and legs, taking care to uncover only one section of skin at a time to avoid chilling her. Rinse off the soap with a wet washcloth, and pat dry.

3. Gently cleanse the baby's genitals. Be careful not to get soap on a newly circumcised penis. For a girl, wipe the vulva from front to back.
4. Wash your baby's bottom last. Rinse with a wet washcloth.
5. If you want to wash your baby's hair, put a dab of shampoo on the wet washcloth. Cradle your baby over a basin or tub, supporting her head and spine with your arm, and use your free hand to lather and rinse her hair. When you're finished, pull the hood over her head, and pat her hair dry. Just like the rest of us, babies quickly lose heat through their heads.

Unless your baby has cradle cap (page 365), it isn't necessary to shampoo her hair more than twice a week.

When your baby is ready to plunge into deeper waters, such as the sink, a baby bathtub, or the regular bathtub (with you in it), the same basic rules apply. The difference is that your baby will be naked for the entire bath and will be mostly submerged in warm water. You'll still need to support your baby's back and neck; keep one hand on the baby even if the tub is designed to support the baby for you.

Once your baby can sit up on her own or can do so with minimal help, you will be able to move her into a full-size tub. For an easier transition, and to free up your hands, you'll probably want to invest in a plastic bath seat, with a safety belt, that sticks by suction to the bottom of the tub. This will help your baby stay safely upright. Whether or not you use such a seat, however, you should never leave the baby during her bath, even for one moment.

Caring for Your Baby's Skin

Your baby's skin is sensitive, so don't blame yourself if his little body suddenly turns red, flaky, or bumpy. But do learn to identify and treat these common infant conditions.

BABY ACNE

Small red or white bumps, typically on the face, sometimes surface around four to five weeks. The condition will resolve itself, usually in a matter of weeks. Meanwhile, keep in mind that harsh detergents or spit-up can exacerbate the problem. Wash your newborn's face with plain water, and launder her clothing and linens in a mild laundry product such as Ivory Snow or Dreft (regular detergents can leave a chemical residue). Avoid using any fabric softener or dryer sheets.

DIAPER RASH

When urine and feces irritate the skin, the result is an angry, red rash that can make your infant very uncomfortable. To treat diaper rash, increase air circulation by closing the diaper loosely or using a larger size. When feasible, let the baby go without a diaper for a spell; lay him on his tummy with an open diaper underneath him and his naked bottom exposed to the air. A couple of hours of this treatment each day are ideal. If the weather is warm, have him lie naked in a shady spot outdoors.

It's essential to keep the affected area clean and dry. This means changing the baby's diaper often and, during diaper changes, washing his bottom with warm water and patting it dry. Don't use soap or baby wipes; they could exacerbate the rash.

Before putting on a fresh diaper, create a protective barrier between the irritants and your baby's skin. Cover the rash with a thick ointment such as Aquaphor (my favorite), A+D ointment, Desitin, or Balmex.

If the rash doesn't clear up within a few days, or if blisters or pustules appear, consult your baby's doctor.

CRADLE CAP

If you notice scaly patches on your infant's head, chances are it is *cradle cap*. This form of eczema affects up to half of all babies. Although it may look unsightly, it won't cause your baby any discomfort. To get rid of it, you can rub a little mineral oil or petroleum jelly on the affected area and wait an hour for the scales to loosen. Then wash your baby's hair with a mild baby shampoo. Repeat this daily until the condition clears, which usually takes about a week. If the cradle cap is severe, your baby's doctor may recommend a medicated shampoo. He or she may even prescribe a cortisone cream or lotion to apply to your baby's head.

TRIMMING YOUR BABY'S NAILS

A newborn's nails may look flimsy, but they are surprisingly sharp. To keep your infant from scratching herself, here's what you'll need to do:

For the first few weeks, it may be easiest to use an emery board to whittle down the nails. Some moms peel off the excess nail with their teeth or fingers.

After the nails thicken a bit, baby nail clippers or high-quality nail scissors with rounded tips should do the trick. To avoid catching the skin, press downward on the finger pad before cutting. Follow the nail's natural curve, taking care to leave a thin white rim behind. Cutting straight across would result in sharp corners. If, despite your best efforts, you end up with jagged edges, you can round them out with an emery board.

Keep in mind that most parents—no matter how cautious—will occasionally nick the skin during a trim. If this happens, don't panic. Your baby's pain will be short-lived. And you can quickly stop any bleeding by wrapping the finger in a tissue or cotton ball and applying gentle pressure.

Fingernails grow quickly. Expect to trim them at least once a week. Toenails usually require less maintenance. Cutting them twice a month should suffice.

If your baby squirms or protests while you're trimming her nails, try cutting them while she is sleeping, or have your partner do it while you are feeding the baby.

DAD'S CORNER

You are a parent! Even though you knew it was going to happen, nothing could quite prepare you for having a completely new little human in the family. You may feel blessed, overwhelmed, and, quite possibly, terrified. Take heart—people have been raising babies for hundreds of thousands of years. Babies are natural, and parenting is natural. But even the most natural of things, such as walking, can take practice. If you spent time babysitting or helping with siblings when you were younger, much of baby care may be second nature for you. If not, don't panic! Skills for holding, calming, and feeding your wonderful child are definitely within your reach.

Be Proactive. Parenting and its rewards have a simple, causal relationship: The more you give, the more you get—from your child, from your mate, from your life. Involved dads report less worry about career achievements, more confidence in unfamiliar situations, and higher overall satisfaction with life. In other words, caring for a baby is good for you! Do respect your mate's need for solitary time with your infant, but make sure you have as much direct contact with the baby as your circumstances allow. Be as efficient as you can at work if this allows you to get home earlier. Even doing little things like changing a diaper while you sing to the baby helps him learn to trust your voice and touch and provides your mate the immeasurable relief of knowing she can depend on you. It is better to do than to worry. You will be amazed at what you can accomplish.

Be a Team Player. A mother is hard-wired for baby care. She wakes easily at night, her milk lets down when her baby cries, her uterus contracts when the child sucks her breast, and she often instinctively knows what her child's needs are. You cannot compete with her bio-psychological connection, and there is no reason to try. You have a most precious gift to offer. Although you may sleep through most of the night feedings, you can help your partner by doing a nighttime diaper change or burping or rocking the baby if she fusses. Even though my husband, Ray, awoke early in the morning for surgery, he coveted his nighttime routine of cradling Alexander in our rocking chair. This was their special time together, when the rest of the world was quiet.

Through diligence, observation, and time with your newborn, your special parenting style will assert itself. Many dads find that their lesser physiological involvement actually seems to help their parenting, by making them easygoing and able to roll with the baby's moods.

Ensure that Mom has what she needs most—good food, plenty of liquids, and assistance with the shopping, meal preparation, and the management of company. If you are able to stay home during the first couple of weeks after the baby's birth, the transition will be smoother. You can really get to know your newborn during this period. You and your partner can sleep and do baby care in shifts without your worrying about having to get up in the morning for work.

If you can't take time off work, it will help Mom a great deal to have some assistance from family members or friends when you are at work. They can do a load of laundry, make a trip to the market, or, at the very least, keep her company. Women have told me they have found helpful even a phone call from someone checking on how Mom and the baby are doing. Best of all might be visits by a postpartum doula, a knowledgeable support person who helps new moms at scheduled times. Ask your childbirth-preparation instructor for information on local postpartum doula services.

Get Support. Your own mental health is crucial to your child and partner. Feeling a little shell-shocked is perfectly natural while acclimating to parenthood, but there are things that you can and should do to help yourself. For starters, don't try to be the Rock of Gibraltar. Let yourself blow off steam outside the home—by going for a run, maybe, or taking a drive with the radio blasting. More helpful still is to find like-minded parents with whom you can share your concerns. You may want others' opinions on questions such as "Why does the baby ignore me after I've been away for a trip?" and "Where did sex go?" It really helps to have a sounding board to whom you aren't married, whether it's a formal support group, family members, or co-workers with kids. These people can help you develop your personal parenting style.

There is no rule that says Dad has to be only a provider and a last-ditch babysitter. The possibilities and rewards of fatherhood are limitless.

THE END OF THE POSTPARTUM PERIOD

Officially, the postpartum period is six weeks after the birth of the baby. During this time, the body gradually returns to its pre-pregnant state. For some women, the process takes less time; for others, more.

The emotional adaptation to motherhood can take at least as long as the time of physical adjustment. I remember that it took me about a month to really feel like a mother. I would sometimes have to pinch myself when I thought, "I'm sure Alexander's real mother will come back soon." Remember that you are still going through an enormous transition. It takes time to integrate motherhood into your identity.

By the time your baby is about one month old, however, you will probably feel a bit more comfortable as a new mom. Your body has done most of its healing, and you and your baby may have developed daily routines. Your baby will have lost the cone head, wrinkles, and scrunched-up face that he may have had at birth. He's gaining control of his body and beginning to move his arms and legs in smooth, steady rhythms. He is much more proficient at grasping and kicking. He has probably begun smiling at you. If he is exceptionally strong, he may even lift his head when he is lying down, hold it steady when he is upright, and follow moving objects with his eyes. He responds to your voice with his body, by moving slowly and rhythmically when you talk to him quietly and gently, and faster when your voice gets animated and intense. New sounds show up in his vocal repertoire. Besides crying, he is beginning to coo and gurgle.

When your baby is hungry, he wants to be fed immediately, and he lets you know with a loud, grouchy cry. When he's wet or sleepy, he expresses those feelings immediately. Your baby lives moment to moment, and his needs at any given moment determine his response to the world. You can probably recognize some of the different needs by his different cries. When you have met all his basic needs for comfort, your baby is ready to play and interact with you. His growing focus on you, and his response to you, will get more exciting every day.

Afterword

ONE OF MY FAVORITE SONGS, by John Mayer, has a line that says, "Girls become lovers who turn into mothers, so, mothers, be good to your daughters, too." This resonates with me because everything in this book concerns the parents that you will become, or already are. When I was pregnant, a close friend who has three children said to me, "Don't wish away your pregnancy or those first sleep-deprived months. One day, you'll wish for them back." This is so true. I love each stage of Alexander's growth, but some days, I wish he still had tiny feet.

Although the parent-child relationship is always complicated, it is also the most fundamental human bond. I would like to share with you a few stories about this bond. The stories were sent to me by people from all over the world. Not everyone has warm feelings about their own parents, and bad feelings about one's own parents can make the experience of becoming a mother or father bittersweet. The stories I share here are positive ones, because a happy parent-child bond is what I hope for you. Some of these stories are humorous, and some are poignant. What ties them all together is the shining thread of love.

ABOUT MOMS

"As I grew up watching my mother, I saw that it was possible to give of myself without giving up myself. Now, as I look ahead to becoming a mother and taking on a job that she made look so easy, I am in awe of what she accomplished and the person that she is. My mother is a writer, and I am a mathematician. She is graceful, and I am a bit clumsy. She is disciplined, and I am absent-minded. She is wise, and I am only beginning to comprehend how much I have to learn."

—Barbara

"Often, as I was coming home from school, my mom was going to work. By the time her shift was over, I was already asleep. But she had every other Friday off, and those Friday nights were girls' night out. We'd go shopping and out to dinner, and spend time with only each other."

—Julie

"When I was six years old and my brother was eleven, my mom left my father. Only now that I have a child do I understand where she found the strength to do it. She worked two, sometimes three, jobs to keep us fed and clothed, and she still managed to spend a lot of time with us. I don't remember ever feeling that we had less than any other children."

—Lanie

"My mom would take me on nature hikes. We would find animal tracks in the drying mud, cast them with plaster, and then go back to my wildlife encyclopedias and figure out what creature had left them. It was wildly exciting. She would point out flowers and plants along the trail, and we'd taste the edible ones. Did you know that miner's lettuce tastes like pineapples? At nightfall, we would lie on our backs on the broad expanse of lawn and she would tell me stories about the constellations, as we'd wish on falling stars."

—Joy

"When my young body was changing and becoming so obviously different from my brothers', my mother held me tight. When I was hurting and needing her, she wrapped her arms around me. She watched and kept near as I struggled against her, trying to find my own place. She often told me of her dreams for me, but was never disappointed by my choice to follow my own road."

—Monica

"There was nothing I loved more than rolling down the back lawn just after Dad had mowed it. And nothing I wanted more than to roll down it stark naked. All through my childhood, I'd fantasized about doing this. Never was allowed to, though. It wasn't done.

One hot July night when I was thirteen, I begged my mother for the ump-teenth time to let me take off my clothes so I could roll, newborn-nude, down the hill in the fragrant, fresh-mown grass. More than 30 years later, I still remember Mom's reaction. She paused. She looked out the window. She looked at me. She looked back out the window. It was sooooo hot. She thinned her lips and nodded her head involuntarily, as if coming to some momentous decision, as if accept-ing that her child was shipping out as a merchant marine. And she said, 'Okay. But first let me turn out the patio light. And you get only one turn.'

I agreed. I was thrilled. I couldn't believe my luck. Quickly I stripped off my pajamas and threw them on the kitchen floor. Mom didn't even make me pick them up! I hurled myself out the door, across the cement patio, and up the hill and flung myself down under the apple tree. I launched my body down the hill.

Over and over, tumbling and rolling, grass spraying and dew spangling, the stars turning into pinwheels as dizziness and giggles swept me up, I became a wild, tangle-topped dandelion blown to pieces by wonder. Mom stood just beyond the open doorway, silhouetted in the light pouring out from the kitchen.

"Come now, quickly," she hissed, holding out a huge bath towel, wrapping me up, hurrying me back into the house, and closing the door, sealing us back inside. She kissed me and told me to go shower away the grass. Little did either of us know, then, that she had opened the kitchen door on the rest of my life that night. When she gave me permission to break the bonds of 'good,' 'nice,' and 'what's not done,' she also gave me the keys to explore my own soul. On my own terms. I'll never forget it."

—Leslie

"Long ago, Mom and I developed a tradition; I no longer remember who started it. The winters in the Midwest can be brutal, but in spring, the world comes back to life. May apples, trilliums, crocuses, and violets are the first flowers to appear. On Mother's Day, Mom and I would hike through the woods behind our house and search for violets. We would select the blue ones, the light lavender, and the deep purple. It was an adventure we shared, just the two of us, without my sisters. We would put some of the flowers in a vase in front of Mom's statue of the Virgin Mary, and the others she would keep on her dresser.

The tradition remains a part of our lives. As an adult, I have sent her live violet plants, dried ones, pictures of violets, and violet-covered cards. When we are together in the spring, we go out together to look for violets. They are a symbol of the thread between us, mother and daughter. Invisible and yet so very, very strong."

—*Tori*

"Becoming a mother in the presence of my own mother is a moment I will never forget. Shortly after my son was born, she sent me a note that said, 'Do you know I love you as much as you love Peter?' I hope she knows that I love her as much as Peter loves me. That's what my card to her will say on my very first Mother's Day."

—*Katie Beth*

AND LET'S NOT LEAVE OUT DADS

"My dad taught me girl things and boy things, but mostly he taught me to believe in myself."

—Elsa

"My father is always bragging about how he is one of the wealthiest men in the world because of the love and joy my sister, my brother, and I have given him."

—Suzanne

"My dad is the greatest because—
- *On the Saturday afternoons that Mom worked, he would make his famous corn-chip pie.*
- *After giving him my big-brown-eyes look, anything was mine for the asking. He later warned my husband about this look!*
- *All babies love to sleep on his belly.*
- *His mesquite-grilled fajitas are out of this world!*
- *He said he didn't like animals, but we caught him baby-talking to our dogs, Gretchen and Daisy.*
- *He cried in front of everybody when my brother, his oldest child, got married.*
- *He cried when my sister's first husband broke her heart.*
- *He cried when I left home to join the Air Force.*
- *He cried when Gretchen and Daisy died.*
- *He's been married to my mom for 45 years."*

—Susie

Glossary

abruptio placenta: see "placental abruption."

AFP test (alpha-feto protein): a test of a maternal blood sample to detect certain genetic birth defects.

afterbirth: the placenta and membranes expelled after the birth of the baby.

afterpains: uterine cramping that occurs after the birth of the baby and the passage of the placenta.

amniocentesis: a test of the amniotic fluid to find out if the baby has any chromosomal defects.

amnion: membrane around the fetus, surrounding the amniotic cavity.

amniotic fluid: the "water" around the baby in the uterus.

analgesic: a drug that diminishes pain.

anemia: any condition in which the blood is lacking in red blood cells or the oxygen-transporting protein hemoglobin.

anesthetic: a drug that removes pain.

anterior presentation: also called occiput presentation, this is the position of the baby at birth when he or she is facing the mother's tailbone. This is the optimal presentation for a vaginal birth.

Apgar score/test: a basic assessment of the baby's well-being, taken at 1 minute and 5 minutes after birth.

areola: the pinkish or brownish area surrounding the nipple of the breast.

artificial rupture of membranes: the use of a small tool to create an opening in the amniotic sac. Also called "breaking the water bag," this procedure can help increase the strength of labor contractions.

back labor: contractions that are felt primarily in the lower back.

bilirubin: a by-product of a pigment that is formed from hemoglobin (the red blood cells' oxygen-carrier) during the recycling of red blood cells in the liver.

biophysical profile: a test of fetal well-being.

blighted ovum: an egg that is fertilized but fails to develop, resulting in a miscarriage or the need for a D&C.

blood pressure: the pressure exerted by the blood against the walls of blood vessels.

bloody show: the mucus and blood expelled when small capillaries around the cervix break as the cervix softens and dilates shortly before birth.

Braxton-Hicks contractions: normal uterine contractions during pregnancy. They are generally not painful or regular and do not indicate the onset of labor.

breech: a baby who is positioned either bottom-down (frank breech) or feet-down (footling breech) instead of head-down (vertex).

capillaries: the smallest blood vessels.

caput: the soft tissue at the top of the baby's head. During a vaginal birth, this area is frequently felt by the practitioner before the bony structure of the baby's head.

carpal tunnel syndrome: a condition in which pain and weakness occur in the hand and forearm. It is caused by pressure on the carpel nerve of the hand, frequently because of swollen tissue or repetitive movements.

cervix: the opening of the uterus, located at the top of the vagina. When a woman isn't in labor, her cervix feels like the tip of a nose.

cesarean section: birth by way of a surgical incision in the lower abdomen and the uterus.

chlamydia: a sexually transmitted infection, serious if left untreated.

chorioamnionitis: an infection of the placenta and membranes surrounding the baby.

chorion: a membrane of the amniotic sac.

circumcision: the removal of the foreskin of the penis.

cleft palate: a congenital malformation of the roof of the mouth.

colostrum: the milk produced by the breast for the first few days after birth. This milk is high in calories and contains large proportions of antibodies and other elements that protect a baby from disease.

condyloma acuminatum: genital warts, also called venereal warts, which result from a sexually transmitted infection.

constipation: difficulty in passing stools, because they are hard.

cord prolapse: a medical emergency in which the umbilical cord emerges before the baby's head or body and the baby's oxygen supply is cut off. This requires immediate delivery by cesarean section.

corpus luteum: the area in the ovary in which the egg is released and progesterone is produced. Progesterone is needed to maintain a pregnancy.

CPD (cephalopelvic disproportion): a condition in which the baby's head is too large to pass through the mother's pelvis.

cystic fibrosis: an inherited disease primarily affecting the respiratory system.

D&C (dilation and curettage): a medical procedure in which the cervix is opened and an instrument is used to remove tissue on the lining of the uterus.

dilation: the process of the opening of the cervix.

Doppler ultrasound device: an instrument that uses sound waves to detect a fetal heartbeat and intensify its sound.

doula: a person who provides physical and emotional support for a woman and her partner during labor.

Down syndrome: also called trisomy 21, a genetic anomaly in which there is an extra number-21 chromosome. The syndrome is characterized by a variable degree of mental retardation and physical abnormalities.

eclampsia: the most severe maternal condition that can develop from pre-eclampsia. Symptoms are seizures and, sometimes, coma.

ectopic pregnancy: a pregnancy that occurs outside the uterus, most commonly in one of the fallopian tubes.

EDC (estimated date of confinement): estimated date when the baby will be born.

EDD (estimated date of delivery): estimated date when the baby will be born.

edema: swelling, or the accumulation of fluid, in tissue.

effacement: the thinning and shortening of the cervix during late pregnancy and labor.

embryo: the developing fertilized egg from conception through the eighth week of pregnancy.

endometriosis: a condition in which patches of uterine lining grow outside the uterus in the abdominal and pelvic cavities, sometimes causing pain.

endometrium: the lining of the uterus.

engagement: the descent of the presenting part of the baby (usually the head) into the mother's pelvis to the level of the pelvic (ischial) spines. Engagement is sometimes referred to as dropping, or lightening.

engorgement: the filling of a breast with milk to the point that the breast becomes swollen, hard, and tender.

epidural anesthesia: the injection of anesthetic medication into the space just outside the spinal membrane to remove most or all sensation in the lower body.

episiotomy: an incision made in the perineum during delivery of the baby to widen the vaginal opening and possibly prevent tearing.

estrogen: a hormone produced primarily in the ovaries during a woman's menstrual cycle and during pregnancy. Estrogen causes the development of female characteristics.

external fetal monitor (EFM): a device by which the baby's heart rate is tracked and recorded through straps placed on the mother's abdomen during labor or in the last trimester of pregnancy.

external version: a procedure in which a practitioner presses his or her hands against the mother's abdomen to turn the baby from a breech to a vertex (head-down) position.

fallopian tube: one of two narrow tubes in a woman's body through which an egg passes from an ovary to the uterus.

false labor: prelabor contractions that can be confused with actual labor because they are frequent and continual, but they do not dilate the cervix. Also called prodromal labor, these contractions are frequently caused by dehydration.

fetal fibronectin (fFN): a protein that is produced during pregnancy and that, if seen in vaginal secretions, may indicate a higher risk of preterm labor.

fetus: the unborn baby from the end of the eighth week of pregnancy until birth.

fibroid: a slow-growing, benign (noncancerous) growth in the uterus.

folic acid: a B vitamin that aids in the prevention of spina bifida.

fontanel: one of two soft areas between a baby's skull plates that allow the head to mold to fit through the mother's pelvis.

footling breech: a baby whose presenting part is a foot and leg.

forceps: a medical instrument used to aid in the delivery of the baby's body during birth.

foremilk: the thin breast milk that a baby receives at the beginning of a feeding.

frank breech: a baby whose presenting part is the buttocks.

fraternal twins: twins that develop from two separate eggs.

fundus: the top of the uterus. **general anesthesia:** anesthesia that causes a person to become unconscious and unable to feel pain during surgery or another medical procedure.

gestation: pregnancy.

gestational diabetes: a condition in which the mother's blood sugar is abnormally elevated during pregnancy.

glucose tolerance test: a laboratory test for gestational diabetes. The test evaluates how the body breaks down sugar in the blood.

gonorrhea: a sexually transmitted disease.

group B streptococcus (GBS): a bacterium that can cause a blood infection in a newborn baby. A woman who is a carrier of this bacterium should receive preventive antibiotics during her labor.

hCG (human chorionic gonadotropin): a hormone that supports the developing embryo and placenta.

hemorrhage: sudden, heavy bleeding.

hemorrhoids: swollen veins in the rectum.

high-risk pregnancy: a pregnancy in which either the mother or the baby has a potentially serious medical condition or is otherwise at risk for developing complications.

hind milk: the rich, thick breast milk that the baby receives at the end of a feeding.

HSG (hysterosalpingogram): a test to evaluate the condition of the uterus and fallopian tubes.

hypertension: high blood pressure.

hysterectomy: the surgical removal of the uterus.

identical twins: twins developing from a single egg that divides into two identical embryos after fertilization.

incompetent cervix: a condition in which a woman's cervix prematurely dilates, often resulting in a miscarriage or premature delivery.

induction of labor: the process of starting labor artificially, through artificial rupture of the membranes, administration of oxytocin, or other means.

infant jaundice: a condition in which the baby's skin and mucous membranes become yellow as a result of slow breakdown of excess red blood cells.

insulin: a hormone secreted in the pancreas that regulates the amount of glucose in the blood. A deficiency results in diabetes.

intramuscular: given into a muscle, as an injected medication.

intrauterine growth retardation (IUGR): a condition in which fetal growth is behind schedule.

intrauterine pressure catheter (IUPC): a device inserted into the uterus to measure the strength of uterine contractions during labor.

intravenous (IV): given into a vein, such as fluid or medication passed through a needle or tube.

Kegel: a strengthening exercise of the perineum and pelvic floor; done by repeatedly tightening and releasing the vaginal muscles.

lactation: the production of milk.

lanugo: the fine, downy hair that covers a baby in the uterus.

letdown reflex: the process in which milk begins to flow through the milk ducts, usually in response to the baby's sucking.

lightening: also called engagement, the descent of the baby into the mother's pelvis during the latter part of pregnancy.

linea negra: a dark line that extends from a woman's navel to the top of the pubic bone during pregnancy. This change in skin pigment is caused by pregnancy hormones.

LMP (last menstrual period): the first day of a woman's most recent menstrual period. This date is commonly used to calculate the baby's due date.

local anesthesia: the injection of anesthetic medication to numb a small, select area of the body.

lochia: the blood that passes from the placental attachment after birth, in what resembles a long and heavy menstrual period.

low-lying placenta: a placenta that is positioned on the lower uterine wall, near the cervix.

mastitis: an infection in the breast tissue during lactation.

meconium: the baby's initial bowel movements. The stool is greenish black, tarry, and sticky.

membranes: amniotic sac, or bag of waters.

miscarriage: the loss of a pregnancy before the baby could survive outside the womb.

misoprostol: a synthetic prostaglandin in the form of a tablet, which is often placed in the cervix to help soften and efface it before oxytocin is administered to induce labor contractions.

molar pregnancy: a pregnancy in which a fertilized egg fails to develop, but abnormal tissue grows. A D&C is frequently needed to remove the tissue.

molding: the temporary elongation of the baby's head as it moves through the mother's pelvis.

mucous plug: the collection of mucus that is sometimes formed within the cervix. The plug sometimes passes out of the vagina just before labor begins.

multigravida: a woman who has been pregnant two or more times.

multipara: a woman who has given birth more than once.

neonate: a newborn baby.

neural tube: the part of the embryo that develops into the baby's brain and spinal cord.

non-stress test: a test of fetal well-being, performed during the last trimester of pregnancy, in which accelerations of the baby's heart rate are measured over a specific period of time.

nuchal translucency screening: a fetal test done by ultrasound that can help determine a baby's risk of heart defects, Down syndrome, and other chromosomal abnormalities.

oligohydramnios: a deficiency of amniotic fluid around the baby.

ovaries: female reproductive organs that produce eggs and the hormones estrogen and progesterone.

ovulation: the ripening and discharge of one or more eggs from an ovary.

oxytocin: a pituitary hormone that stimulates uterine contractions during labor and triggers the release of breast milk.

pap test: also called a pap smear, this is a test to detect cancerous or precancerous cells of the cervix.

perinatal: the time period around childbirth, from about six weeks before to about four weeks after.

perinatologist: an obstetrician specializing in high-risk pregnancy.

perineum: the area between the vagina and the anus.

phenylketonuria (PKU): a genetic disorder in which the baby's body is unable to metabolize the essential amino acid phenylalanine, which is found in particular foods. The condition can be treated through a special diet. If left untreated, PKU can lead to mental retardation.

Pitocin: synthetic oxytocin, administered to initiate labor contractions, increase their strength, or prevent excessive blood loss after birth.

placenta previa: a placenta that is positioned at the base of the uterus, covering the cervix. This condition necessitates a cesarean birth.

placenta: the organ that develops during pregnancy to supply nutrients and oxygen to the fetus through the umbilical cord.

placental abruption: the separation of the placenta from the uterine wall before the birth of the baby. The separation can result in severe bleeding in the mother and lack of oxygen for the baby.

polyhydramnios: an excessive amount of amniotic fluid.

posterior presentation: the position of the baby at birth when he or she is facing away from the mother's tailbone. This position frequently causes back labor.

postmature baby: a baby whose gestation lasts more than 42 weeks or whose placenta shows signs of having exceeded the period of optimal function.

preeclampsia : also known as toxemia, a dangerous condition of pregnancy that, if left untreated, can develop into eclampsia. Symptoms include general swelling and fluid retention, sudden and excessive weight gain, high blood pressure, and protein in the urine. The exact cause is unknown.

premature baby: a baby born before 36 to 37 weeks of gestation.

presentation: the position of the baby for birth, described according to the part of the baby's body that will first emerge from the vagina.

preterm labor: labor that begins before 36 to 37 weeks of gestation.

primagravida: a woman experiencing her first pregnancy.

primapara: a woman who has given birth once.

progesterone : a female hormone that is produced by the corpus luteum during the menstrual cycle and by the placenta to maintain a pregnancy.

prolactin: a pituitary hormone that stimulates lactation.

prostaglandin: a fatty acid that mimics the action of particular hormones.

quad screen test: a test of a mother's blood to screen for specific birth defects and genetic disorders.

quickening: the first fetal movements that the mother feels.

regional anesthesia: medication that numbs a select, large area of the body. An example is epidural anesthesia.

Rh factor: a group of antigens (antibody-producing) substances present in most people's red blood cells.

Rh sensitivity: a condition in which the body of an Rh-negative mother creates harmful antibodies to her unborn baby's red blood cells.

RhoGAM: a trade name for Rh immune globulin, which is injected into an Rh-negative pregnant woman to prevent hemolytic disease in her newborn.

round ligament: one of two ligaments supporting the uterus.

sciatica: pain caused by pressure on the sciatic nerve, which extends from the back of the hip and buttocks down the leg.

sonogram: an image produced through ultrasound.

spider veins: small, capillary veins that become visible during pregnancy, most commonly on legs.

spina bifida: a congenital abnormality in which a part of the spinal cord or spinal membranes protrudes through an opening in the spinal column; results in partial or total paralysis.

spinal block: used primarily for surgery, the injection of anesthetic directly into the spinal fluid; results in temporary numbness and paralysis of the lower body.

spontaneous abortion: miscarriage.

station: the location of the baby in the pelvis, from -4, the top of the pelvis, to 0, engagement, to +4, birth.

stillbirth: the death of a baby during the third trimester of pregnancy.

stretch marks: white, pink, or reddish streaks on the skin, usually on the breasts, thighs, or abdomen, which result from rapid expansion of skin in the area where the marks occur. The marks frequently appear during pregnancy and are most common in light-skinned people.

surfactant: the sudsy substance in the baby's lungs that develops at approximately 35 to 36 weeks' gestation. The substance lubricates the lining of the lungs to allow the infant to breathe normally at birth and afterward.

Tay-Sachs disease: an inherited disease that occurs among some people of Jewish descent and that causes mental and physical disability.

terbutaline: a smooth-muscle relaxant that is used to decrease or eliminate preterm contractions.

thalassemia major: a genetic condition that occurs among people of Mediterranean and Southeast Asian descent and that results in severe anemia.

thalassemia minor: a mild form of thalassemia.

toxemia: preeclampsia.

toxoplasmosis: a disease, harmful to a fetus, that is caused by a parasite and transmitted through undercooked meat and the feces of infected animals, especially cats.

transition: in active labor, the period when uterine contractions are the strongest and longest and the cervix dilates from about 7 to about 10 centimeters.

transverse: a baby's horizontal position in the mother's abdomen.

trimester: a period of about 13 weeks at the beginning, middle, or end of gestation.

ultrasound: high-frequency sound waves, which can be used to create an image of the baby in the uterus.

uterus: also called the womb, the hollow, muscular organ of the pelvic region in which the baby develops and grows before birth.

vacuum extractor: a suction device used to aid in the delivery of the baby's head.

varicose veins: veins, especially in the legs, that have become swollen from a structural defect or increased pressure or blood flow.

VBAC (vaginal birth after cesarean): vaginal birth by a woman who has previously had a baby by cesarean.

vena cava: one of two major blood vessels that carry circulating blood back to the heart.

vernix: the thick, creamy coating that protects a baby's skin in the amniotic fluid and often is present at birth.

vertex: the baby's head, or the baby's head-down position in the mother's body.

Appendix A

LISTS, LISTS, AND MORE LISTS

THIS APPENDIX CONDENSES advice from throughout the chapters of this book. You may find it helpful to view this material as it is organized here, by topic. Then, for more detail, you can refer back to the chapter that each list came from.

CHOOSING YOUR CHILDBIRTH OPTIONS

Once you find out that you are pregnant, you face a lot of homework in planning your baby's birth. The following lists summarize some of the essential questions to ask as you look for the childbirth options that will work best for you.

Choosing a Birth Facility

- How far is the facility from your home?
- Is one-on-one care provided throughout labor? What is the nurse-to-patient ratio?
- Are there CNMs (certified nurse-midwives) on staff?
- Who is allowed to be with you in labor? During the birth itself? What if you have a cesarean birth?
- Are there any policies regarding the use of independent doulas (labor-support persons)?

- Will you give birth in the same room that you labor in? Can you look at the rooms?
- Does the facility have policies about the use of medical procedures such as fetal monitoring (intermittent or continuous) and the administration of intravenous (IV) fluids, or does the individual practitioner determine when and how these procedures are used?
- Will you be allowed to move about freely during labor?
- Do the rooms have showers, whirlpool baths, or other bathtubs?
- Will you be allowed to eat and drink during labor?
- Is there an anesthesiologist on staff at all times?
- Is epidural anesthesia (page 298) available? Is there any restriction on when you can receive it?
- What is the epidural rate?
- Will the baby be able to stay in your room after the birth, or will the baby be taken to a nursery?
- Can you see the operating room where cesareans are performed? If you have a cesarean, can the baby stay with you afterward?
- What is the cesarean rate?
- If you or the baby requires special care, can both of you stay at the facility, or will you be transferred to another hospital?
- Does the hospital have a neonatal intensive-care unit (NICU)? If so, what level of care does it provide?
- What is the policy on breastfeeding? Can you specify that the baby not receive bottles of formula or sugar water?
- Is there a lactation consultant on staff?
- Does the hospital or birth center offer prenatal and parenting classes? Are there new-parent support groups?

Choosing a Practitioner

- How long is a typical office visit?
- How many births does the practitioner, or group of practitioners, manage each month?
- What are the practitioner's feelings and practices regarding fetal monitoring, epidurals, and other medications in labor? How about episiotomy, cesarean birth, and breastfeeding?
- In what situations does the practitioner induce labor? Is labor routinely induced if it doesn't begin spontaneously before 41 or 42 weeks?
- What percentage of the practitioner's clients give birth by cesarean? What is the cesarean rate for the entire practice?
- At what point in labor does the practitioner arrive?
- If the practitioner is a doctor, does the practice include certified nurse-midwives?
- Will you meet everyone in a group practice before the baby is born?
- If you have a question or a problem, how do you reach the doctor or midwife?

Choosing a Childbirth Preparation Class

- Who sponsors the classes—the hospital or birth center where you'll deliver, a separate organization, or an individual?
- What are the instructor's credentials? Is the person affiliated with any organization?
- Does the class advocate a particular philosophy? If so, what is it? Does the approach seem practical and objective?
- What topics are covered in the class?
- How does this class differ from others offered in the area?
- How many couples are in each class?
- Can you bring more than one support person? Can you come alone?
- Where is the class held?

- How many meetings are in each series of classes, and how long does each meeting last? Are there different options for class times, such as evenings, weekends, or all day?
- What is the cost for the class? Will your health insurance cover any of the cost?
- Do you need to bring anything with you?

Discussing Labor with Your Practitioner

- Will your practitioner definitely attend your delivery? If not, who might take his or her place? Will you be able to meet the substitute practitioner before you give birth?
- At what point in labor should you call your practitioner? When should you go to the hospital or birth center?
- If your water bag breaks or if you go past your due date, how long will your practitioner wait before inducing your labor?
- If your labor must be induced, what method will be used?
- Will you have continuous fetal monitoring, or can it be intermittent? Does your hospital or birth center offer telemetry monitoring or use a hand-held device?
- Will you be automatically subjected to any medical procedures, such intravenous (IV) fluids, the insertion of an IV injection port (in case IV fluids are needed later), or an episiotomy? Or will these be done only if necessary?
- Who can be with you during your labor and birth?
- Will you be able to walk around, change positions, and labor in a shower, regular bath, or whirlpool bath?
- Will you be able to eat and drink in labor?
- What are your practitioner's views on pain medications and anesthesia in labor? Are there any rules regarding how far along you need to be in your labor before using them? Do others in the practice have different rules?
- What are your practitioner's criteria in deciding that a cesarean birth is necessary?

- If you need to have a cesarean, can you elect to be awake and have your partner or other support person with you?
- After the birth, does the baby stay with you or go to the nursery? Can you choose? If the baby does go to the nursery, how long will she need to stay there?
- Can you choose to keep your baby with you continuously after birth, even at night?
- Can your partner stay overnight with you after the baby is born? What sleeping accommodations will be provided for your partner?
- If you are breastfeeding, can you request that your baby not receive any sugar water or formula?
- Will someone help you get started with breastfeeding? Is there a lactation consultant on staff?
- How long can you expect to remain in the hospital or birth center after a vaginal birth? A cesarean birth? Can you go home early, if you choose?

CARING FOR YOUR OWN BODY

Amid the myriad duties of preparing your home and your world for a new baby, you need to take special care of yourself, too. The following lists summarize some of the best advice for tending to your own needs while you are pregnant.

Twelve Ways to Survive Morning Sickness

- Soothe your stomach with carbonated drinks such as colas and ginger ale.
- Eat smaller, more frequent meals, five to six a day.
- Eat something even before you get out of bed in the morning, if necessary.
- Eat anything that appeals to you, including milk shakes, ice cream, pasta, or other high-calorie foods.
- Stay away from spicy or fried foods and smells that make you queasy.
- Take your prenatal vitamin with your largest meal.
- Sip mint tea, or smell a freshly cut lemon.
- Try to slow down.
- Brush your teeth gently and quickly, and don't brush your tongue. If the taste of the toothpaste bothers you, try switching brands.
- Try motion-sickness bands.
- Try acupuncture.
- Get plenty of fresh air.

Seven Ways to Survive Prescribed Bed Rest

1. *Set up your space.* Put a cooler at your bedside. In the morning before your partner goes to work, have him put your lunch, snacks, and plenty of water and other cold drinks in it. Have him set up a TV and DVD player in front of your perch, and a table at your side.

On it, you'll keep the following items:

- Any medicine you must take
- This book
- Two nonpregnancy books, different enough to suit your changing moods
- A telephone and phone numbers
- An MP3 player with music and audio books or a CD player and recordings
- A calendar
- A laptop computer with Internet access
- The daily newspaper

2. *Start a project.* Design your baby's birth announcement; even address and stamp the envelopes. Learn a new hobby, like knitting or crocheting. Start a journal; this may be hard to believe, but later on, it will be fun to look back on this time. Study a foreign language through books, recordings, and the Internet.

3. *Socialize.* Put the word out to family and friends that you would like visitors—just to hang out, to watch a movie, or to play cards. Write letters to family and friends. Send e-mail or instant messages to keep in touch with folks.

4. *Amuse yourself.* Get good at solitaire. Subscribe to a Hollywood rubbish magazine. Work the newspaper's daily crossword or sudoku puzzle. Paint your toenails and fingernails, ask a friend to do this, or schedule an in-home professional pedicure.

5. *Pamper yourself.* Schedule an in-home weekly massage, if you can afford it, or enlist Dad. If friends ask how they can help, have them do a load of laundry or bring you a home-cooked meal. Feel free to nap!

6. *Mark off each day of your pregnancy on your calendar.*

7. Always remember that you are doing the important job of helping to keep your baby safe inside.

A Good, Basic Relaxation Exercise

Taking one area at a time, from toes to head, contract the muscles of your body for a count of two, and then slowly let the muscles go limp and loose, paying attention to the feeling of releasing tension. Here is a sequence you can follow.

1. Pull your toes down, and then relax.
2. Pull your toes up, and then relax.
3. Turn your ankles out, and then relax.
4. Bend your knees slightly, and then relax.
5. Extend your left leg out, and then relax.
6. Extend your right leg out, and then relax.
7. Tighten your buttocks, and then relax.
8. Tighten your pelvic-floor muscles (do a Kegel), and then relax.
9. Expand your abdominal muscles, and then relax.
10. Make fists, and then relax.
11. Extend your fingers, and then relax.
12. Bend your wrists down, and then relax.
13. Bend your wrists up, and then relax.
14. Straighten your elbows, and then relax.
15. Raise your shoulders, and then relax.
16. Squeeze your chest muscles, and then relax.
17. Expand your chest, and then relax.
18. Pull your shoulder blades forward, and then relax.
19. Pull your shoulder blades back, and then relax.
20. Arch your lower back, and then relax.
21. Bend your neck forward, and then relax.
22. Tighten your jaw, and then relax.
23. Raise your eyebrows, and then relax.
24. Squeeze your facial muscles, and then relax.

Now take another deep, slow breath, and slowly exhale. Lie still for a few more moments to be mindful of the wonder of your child and to enjoy the sensation of full relaxation. Be aware of what it feels like to be limp, loose, and heavy. Just as tension can spread throughout your body, so can relaxation.

Exercise for Visualizing and Relaxing During Labor

1. Find your focal point, or close your eyes.
2. Take your initial cleansing breath, and begin either slow or modified breathing.
3. Imagine that you are climbing up a hill, getting up to the top, and then coming back down. Visualize yourself climbing up the hill as the contraction gets stronger, reaching the top of the hill as the contraction peaks, and climbing down as the contraction fades. If your partner is with you, have him tell you about your climb and descent as he times your imaginary 1-minute contraction. Take 20 seconds or so to climb up the mountain, 10 or 15 at the top, and another 20 as you descend.
4. Finish with another deep, cleansing breath.
5. Repeat the exercise using the second breathing pattern for active labor.

LABOR: THE REAL THING

Recognizing true labor, and having a variety of tools to cope with it, will help you have a happy, healthy, and unforgettable birth experience.

The 5-1-1 Recipe for Knowing When to Go to the Hospital

When your contractions follow the 5-1-1 Recipe, you are very likely beginning active labor.

The 5-1-1 Recipe means—

- Your contractions are coming **5** minutes apart.
- They are lasting **1** minute each.
- They have been this way for **1** full hour.
- *And most importantly: You aren't able to talk or walk during a contraction.*
- It is time to go to the hospital or birth center or have your midwife come to you.

Ways to Use Focus as a Coping Tool in Labor

- Close your eyes and concentrate on some image: a soothing scene, a color, the spots of light you see when your eyes are closed, or your body as a flower opening to give birth to the baby.
- Look for an object or a mark on the floor or wall one to two feet away. Keep your eyes on that spot throughout your entire contraction.
- Pay attention to the sound of your breath. Hear yourself inhale. Hear yourself exhale. If you like, vocalize as you exhale.
- Focus on your contraction. Mentally follow it as it begins, climbs, peaks, descends, and ends.

Breathing for Labor

SLOW BREATHING

1. Take a cleansing breath as each contraction begins.
2. Breathe slowly and deeply, at half your normal respiration rate, and preferably in through your nose and out through your mouth.
3. Take a cleansing breath at the end of the contraction.

MODIFIED BREATHING

1. Take a cleansing breath as each contraction begins.
2. Breathe fast, at twice your normal respiration rate, and preferably in through your nose and out through your mouth.
3. Take a cleansing breath at the end of the contraction.

Ways to Offer Your Laboring Partner Support

1. Assist her in maintaining a relaxed body and attitude. Help her to be as loose and limp as possible.
2. Encourage her to walk and to change positions frequently. Alternate walking with rest periods.
3. In early (latent) labor, help distract her from her contractions. Walk in the park, go to a movie, or even go shopping.
4. Encourage her to drink liquids frequently.
5. Talk to her softly and lovingly during her contractions. If each

of her contractions lasts about the same length of time, use your watch to let her know when she is halfway done. If she is on a uterine monitor, you can tell when the contraction is starting, peaking, and ending by watching the graph line. Knowing that a contraction is nearly over can help her get through it.

6. Help her with her breathing techniques and concentration.

7. Remind her to deal with just one contraction at a time.

8. Encourage and assist her to shower or bathe. It is wonderful to labor in water!

9. Touch and support her physically during each contraction, unless she prefers not to be touched.

10. Massage her wherever it feels good to her. Apply counter pressure on her lower back. To protect your own back, position yourself close to her, lean in, and use your body weight rather than arm strength to apply pressure.

11. *Occasionally* time and record contractions.

12. Apply balm to her lips if they are getting dry.

13. Praise her often. Remain positive, especially if her confidence is dwindling. Don't let her lose sight of the fact that she will have a baby in her arms soon.

14. Offer her ice chips or juice bars.

15. Wipe her face with cool, wet cloths when she is perspiring.

16. Let her know if you need to leave the room. Try not to leave her alone during contractions unless she requests it.

17. Remind her to pee every hour or so. She may feel only the pressure of the contractions and not realize that her bladder is full.

18. Bring her a blanket and socks if she needs them.

Eight Tips for Massaging a Woman in Labor

1. Work with whatever position she finds most comfortable.
2. Use long, flowing strokes. Stroke from the center of her body downward and outward. For example, to massage her arm, start with her shoulder and slowly move down to her elbow, wrist, and fingers.
3. Stroke slowly—fewer than ten times per minute—to decrease muscle activity rather than stimulate it.
4. Always keep one hand in contact with her skin.
5. Use talcum powder or oil to reduce friction.
6. Keep your touch light enough to relieve tension, but firm enough to avoid tickling. Very light touch can feel to a woman in active labor a bit like a mosquito buzzing in her ear.
7. Use less motion and firmer pressure on her lower back.
8. If she is experiencing back labor, she will probably want firm massage in the lowest part of her back, near her coccyx. Ask her to place your hand on the spot that has the most pressure.

SHOP TILL YOU DROP

Depending on whether you love to shop or not, you may find these lists of the things you need either exciting or odious. In either case, these lists are a good jumping-off point for gathering what you may need for yourself, your partner, and your new arrival.

What You Need for Your New Arrival

FURNISHINGS AND LINENS

- Crib
- Crib mattress
- Bumpers
- Bassinet or cradle
- Three-sided sleeper
- Diaper container
- Portable crib or playpen

- Changing space
- Baby tub
- Tub seat
- Vibrating bouncy chair
- Swing

OUTING EQUIPMENT (FOR LEAVING THE HOUSE)
- Stroller
- Carriage or pram
- Car seat
- Bottles
- Nipples
- Snap-bottom body shirts
- Gowns
- Booties and socks
- Pull-on stretch pants
- One-piece outfits
- Hooded terry-cloth towels
- Sweaters
- Hats
- Snowsuit or bunting outfit
- Receiving blanket
- Diapers
- Wipes
- Wipe warmer
- Burp cloths

ITEMS FOR LATER
- High chair
- Childproofing supplies
- Safety gates

Medical Supplies and Toiletries for Your Baby

- Infant acetaminophen, for fever.
- Alcohol and cotton balls, if your baby's doctor recommends them for the umbilical cord stump.
- Sunscreen, for use only after the first six months.
- Calibrated dropper, for administering medicine.
- Bulb syringe, for clearing a stuffy nose.
- Baby nail clippers or scissors.
- Digital thermometer, for taking the baby's temperature in the rectum, mouth, or armpit.
- Diaper-rash ointment. I prefer Aquaphor, an ointment containing lanolin and mineral oil.
- Petroleum jelly or Aquaphor, to lubricate a rectal thermometer and to protect a newly circumcised penis from urine.
- Baby brush and comb.
- Pedialyte or Ricelyte, for hydration in case the baby has vomiting or diarrhea.
- Activated charcoal, to treat poisoning. Use it only on the recommendation of a physician or poison-control center.
- Baby bath wash or gentle glycerin soap.
- Baby shampoo. Or use baby bath wash instead.

Special Gifts to Request for Your Baby Shower

- Diaper service (one month or more)
- Breast-pump rental
- Lullaby recordings
- Books on infant care
- Books on child growth and development
- Classic picture books or story books
- Towels embroidered with the baby's name
- A handmade quilt or afghan
- Handmade keepsakes, such as a pillow embroidered with the baby's name, a needlepoint pillow, or a cross-stitched plaque

- Gift certificates for dinner out, food delivery, babysitting, house cleaning, or massage (for Mom)
- A homemade dinner, to be served after the baby's birth
- Footprint and handprint kits
- Hand-painted wooden alphabet letters that spell out the baby's name
- A photo album or scrapbook and related supplies

What to Take to the Hospital

FOR MOM

- Bathrobe and slippers
- Basic toiletry items (toothbrush, hairbrush, hair clip or hair band)
- Favorite socks
- Breath spray or breath mints
- Lip balm
- Massage oil
- Massage aid (although your partner's hand will work fine)
- Comfortable pillow (with a case that isn't white, so you don't forget to bring it home)
- Frozen ice or juice bars, or your favorite juice or other cold drink
- Small cooler (if no refrigerator will be available)
- Music player or laptop for music streaming. Check if your birth place has the ability to stream music. If not, you may need to make a playlist.
- Reading material, magazines, laptop, or a deck of cards (especially helpful if you are having your labor induced)
- Nursing bra (if you already have one)
- Extra pair of underpants
- Loose, comfortable clothes for going home (you could wear the same outfit home that you arrive in)

FOR THE PARTNER

- Simple, nourishing snack food
- Basic toiletry items
- Change of clothes (all clothes should be comfortable and easy to move in)
- Swimming suit (in case you want to go into the shower or bath with Mom)
- Phone and battery charger (labeled so that you remember to take it home)
- Video or still camera (if you want to take more detailed photos and videos than with your phone). Hospitals do not allow videos to be taken of medical or surgical procedures, but you can certainly take them of the baby!

FOR THE BABY

- Outfit for the trip home
- Warm blanket (if the weather is cold)
- If you plan on walking home, you can carry your baby in a carrier. If you are driving or taking a ride service home, you'll need to have the base and car seat installed in that vehicle for the trip.

Packing Your Diaper Bag

- At least three disposable or four cloth diapers.
- At least two diaper covers, if you are using cloth diapers.
- A plastic-coated changing pad, either attached to the diaper bag or tucked in separately.
- Two plastic zipper bags.
- Baby wipes.
- Diaper ointment, if your baby has a rash.
- At least two changes of baby clothes.
- An extra sweater, a receiving blanket, or both.
- Nursing pads.
- A hat with a brim or earflaps, depending on the time of year.
- Baby sun block, after the first six months.
- Two extra pacifiers, if your baby uses them.
- Formula, if you are using it.
- One extra empty bottle, if you are formula feeding.
- The phone number for your baby's doctor.

Appendix B

A MONTH-BY-MONTH CHECKLIST OF THINGS TO DO

Before Pregnancy

- Become as healthy as possible and come as close to your ideal weight as possible.
- Get a full medical and gynecological checkup, including a pap smear.
- Be sure your immunizations are up-to-date.
- Begin taking prenatal vitamins that include at least 400 micrograms (mcg) of folic acid.
- Cut down on, or stop, any alcohol, cigarette, or drug intake.

Month One

- Confirm your pregnancy with an at-home pregnancy test.
- Make sure you are eating well and are getting enough rest.
- Stop smoking (for you and your baby).
- Cut out alcohol and drugs, and check with a physician if you are taking prescribed medications. Some are not safe during pregnancy.
- Get used to the idea of being pregnant!

Month Two

- Calculate your due date.
- Investigate your insurance coverage for prenatal care, birth, and baby care.
- Select your practitioner, and schedule your first prenatal appointment.
- Choose a hospital or birthing center.
- Continue eating well, and if you are nauseated, try different strategies to alleviate morning sickness.
- Tell your family and friends about your pregnancy.

Month Three

- Learn about your prenatal testing options, and have the appropriate tests.
- Shop for or borrow maternity clothes. Consider the season during which you will need them most.
- Inform your employer about your pregnancy.

Month Four

- Drink plenty of water every day.
- Try to take a walk each day or to do some other exercise.
- Pre-register at your hospital or birth center.
- Enjoy feeling your baby move for the first time.

Month Five

- Use your prenatal stretching and other exercises to minimize pregnancy discomforts.
- Sign up for childbirth education classes.
- Begin planning your baby's nursery or sleeping area.
- Think about what baby names you are interested in.
- Get a prenatal massage.

Month Six

- Register at a store for you baby shower gifts.
- Select a crib and other baby furniture.
- Interview and choose your baby's pediatrician.
- Check with your insurance company about alerting it to your baby's birth, and be sure that the baby is covered.
- Discuss with your partner whether you will want your son to be circumcised.

Month Seven

- Purchase baby clothes and supplies, and begin setting up your nursery.
- Plan your baby shower.
- Decide how much time you will be taking off when the baby is born, and discuss this with your employer.
- Decide whether you will be breastfeeding, and purchase supplies.
- Select your birth announcements and thank-you notes.
- Organize some simple medical supplies for your baby.
- Investigate where to go for breastfeeding and postpartum support.

Month Eight

- Attend childbirth classes.
- Finish setting up your baby's nursery.
- Have your baby shower.
- Practice labor preparation and relaxation methods.
- Discuss your labor preferences with your practitioner.
- Select whom you would like to be with you in labor.
- Wash all the baby bedding and clothes in a mild laundry soap.
- Prepare your phone list of whom to call once the baby is born.
- Purchase the baby's car seat.

Month Nine

- Pack your suitcase for your birth facility.
- Prepare and freeze some simple meals for the first week after the baby is born.
- Arrange for help during the first weeks after the baby is born.
- Plan for who will care for your home or pets while you are away during your baby's birth.
- Get a pedicure.
- Write your baby shower thank-you notes.
- Install your baby's car seat, and have it checked by an expert (highway patrol or a baby store).

After Your Baby's Birth

- Rest or sleep when your baby sleeps.
- Eat nutritiously, and drink plenty of water.
- Accept help from friends and family.
- Send out your birth announcements.
- Apply for your baby's birth certificate and Social Security number.
- Enjoy your baby!

Appendix C

FOR FURTHER READING

IN CASE YOU WISH TO READ further about pregnancy, childbirth, and babies, I am offering this list of my favorite books, including two for those of you who are trying to conceive but haven't yet. Please know that when you browse in your local library or bookstore you may find other parenting books that speak especially to you.

Infertility Survival Handbook, **by Elizabeth Swire-Falker (Riverhead, 2004)**

Elizabeth Swire-Falker has written an immensely useful and readable book based on her own experience of infertility and years of infertility treatments. Medically well researched, the book is written in the compassionate voice of one who knows how an infertile woman feels.

Riding the Infertility Roller Coaster: A Guide to Educate and Inspire, **by Iris Waichler (Wyatt-Mackenzie, 2006)**

Chock-full of information presented with sensitivity, this book addresses the emotional and physical issues surrounding infertility and treatment for it. The book is helpful not only for couples experiencing infertility but also for their loved ones.

The Girlfriends' Guide to Pregnancy, **2nd Edition, by Vicki Iovine (Pocket, 2007)**

As you have found here in *The Joy of Pregnancy*, having babies is not all serious. This book provides the warmth and comic relief so often missing in books about pregnancy. Vicki Iovine speaks not as a medical professional but as a mother of four babies and a brutally honest, very funny woman. She truly writes in the language of girlfriends.

The Expectant Father: Facts, Tips, and Advice for Dads-to-Be, 3rd Edition, by Armin A. Brott (Abbeville, 2015)

This is a terrific guide for guys. Month by month, it covers the physical and emotional aspects of pregnancy and birth. It also addresses financial concerns and offers practical advice on everything from what Dad is going to see during birth to dealing with being up in the night with the baby. All of this is done with humor and a can-do attitude.

When You're Expecting Twins, Triplets, or Quads: Proven Guidelines for a Healthy Multiple Pregnancy, 3rd Edition, by Barbara Luke, M.D., and Tamara Eberlein (Collins, 2010)

This book is written from both a medical perspective and the personal experience of actual moms of multiples. The authors focus strongly on nutrition but also include a lot of advice on decreasing the odds of complications and managing the wide array of emotions that women pregnant with multiples may feel. The illustrations are simple and clear, and there are even recipes for weight management.

Ina May's Guide to Childbirth, by Ina May Gaskin (Bantam, 2003)

I loved Ina May Gaskin's classic book *Spiritual Midwifery*, and this book is written with the same wisdom and love. More than 2,000 babies have been born at The Farm, the author's home in Summertown, Tennessee, under the care of The Farm's midwives. Ina May Gaskin has unsurpassed knowledge of natural birth and profound respect for labor and a woman's strength. Her stories are a pleasure to read.

The Nursing Mother's Companion, 7th Revised Edition, by Kathleen Huggins, R.N., M.S. (The Harvard Common Press, 2017)

I kept *The Nursing Mother's Companion* right by my rocking chair when Alexander was a baby. Kathleen Huggins's advice is practical, supportive, and extremely reassuring. I found the "survival guides" for each stage of breastfeeding to be invaluable, and the appendix on drug safety excellent. Completely revised and updated on the twentieth anniversary of its publication, this classic guide is still the most helpful breastfeeding book available.

The Preemie Parents' Companion: The Essential Guide to Caring for Your Premature Baby in the Hospital, at Home, and Through the First Years, **by Susan L. Madden (The Harvard Common Press, 2000)**

Having a premature infant is a stressful experience. This book is a comprehensive guide to staying involved in and informed about a preemie's care and coping with medical complications and treatments. Susan Madden guides parents in staying physically and emotionally close to their babies and helps them understand what kind of care they may expect for the baby in the future.

The Baby Book, **Revised Edition by William Sears, M.D. and Martha Sears, R.N. (Little, Brown, & Co., 2013)**

The Baby Book contains valuable information on issues that are not covered in other parenting books. The Sears's philosophy of "attachment parenting" emphasizes breastfeeding, "baby-wearing" (using a sling), and sharing a bed with the baby.

The Girlfriends' Guide to Surviving the First Year of Motherhood, **by Vicki Iovine (Perigee Trade, 1997)**

This book, on managing life with a new baby, provides the same kind of witty advice as *The Girlfriends' Guide to Pregnancy.*

Touchpoints, Birth to 3: Your Child's Emotional and Behavioral Development, **Second Edition, by T. Berry Brazelton, M.D., and Joshua D. Sparrow, M.D. (Da Capo, 2006)**

T. Berry Brazelton is the nation's quintessential pediatrician. His advice is comprehensive, down-to-earth, and reassuring. This book has been my personal guide to understanding the stages of Alexander's growth and behavioral development.

Caring for Your Baby and Young Child: Birth to Age Five, **5th Edition, by the American Academy of Pediatrics (Bantam, 2009)**

This encyclopedic guide is written in the authoritative style of seasoned pediatricians, but it's very easy to read. The medical information is solid, and the simple graphic illustrations are very informative. The first part of the book provides comprehensive parenting information, mostly for the first year. The second half concerns childhood illnesses, immunizations, behavioral problems, and emergency first-aid. I still keep this book close at hand.

Your Baby and Child: From Birth to Age Five, **Revised Edition, by Penelope Leach (Dorling Kindersley, 2010)**

This book explains the pros and cons of various parenting choices and offers practical solutions to common problems. Penelope Leach is very respectful of children, parents, and the family as a whole, and her no-nonsense style is conversational and positive. The book is full of terrific color photographs of children and real families.

The Fourth Trimester Companion, **by Cynthia Gabriel (Harvard Common Press, 2017)**

New mothers so often say that they don't feel prepared for those hours, days, and weeks *after* their baby is born. This is a lovely new book that walks a new mom and her partner through those early days of postpartum recovery and newborn care. It is filled with photographs, lists, and practical suggestions, all in a warm, supportive tone.

Appendix D

HELPFUL ORGANIZATIONS FOR PARENTS AND PARENTS-TO-BE

MANY ORGANIZATIONS in the United States provide information about pregnancy, birth, babies, and breastfeeding. These are some of my favorites.

The Joy of Pregnancy: The Complete, Candid, and Reassuring Resource for Parents-to-be, www.thejoyofpregnancy.com

StorkNet: The Premier Pregnancy and New Parenting Community, www.storknet.com
Talk to others who are experiencing what you are experiencing, and get my answers to your questions.

March of Dimes Resource Center, www.marchofdimes.com
Loads of information on pre-pregnancy, pregnancy, medications, birth defects, and so much more.

International Childbirth Education Association, www.icea.org, (800) 624-4934
Information on childbirth education.

Sidelines: High-Risk Pregnancy and Support Network, www.sidelines.org, (888) 447-4754
Support for high-risk mothers and their families.

Multiples of America (formerly the National Organization of Mothers of Twins Clubs), www.multiplesofamerica.org
Contact this support group early on if you find out that you are expecting twins or more.

Triplets and Us, www.tripletsandus.com
Information and support for parents of twins, triplets, and more.

University of California, San Diego, Pregnancy Drug Hotline, 1-866-626-6847
Information about prescriptive and nonprescriptive drugs that may be harmful to an unborn child.

Centers for Disease Control and Prevention, www.cdc.gov
A wealth of information on pregnancy and medical issues.

National Institutes of Health, www.health.nih.gov
Valuable information on health and medicine.

DONA (Doulas of North America) International, www.dona.org, (888) 788-DONA
Information on labor and postpartum doulas.

La Leche League International, www.llli.org, (877) 452-5324 Mother-to-mother breastfeeding support.

International Lactation Consultant Association, www.ilca.org, (888) 452-2478
Referrals and information on locating a lactation consultant.

Index

Sex
    of baby, 119
    during pregnancy,
        128–130, 136, 232–233
Sexual desire, 129
Shampoo, baby, 218
Sheets, 203
Shellfish, 43–44
Shirts
    baby, 213–214, 361
    maternity, 145
Shoes, 146
Shortness of breath, 258–259
Shorts, 145
Short-term disability, 108
Shoulder hold, 342
Shoulder rolls, 150
Shower gifts, 196–197
Showering, during labor, 276,
    285
Showing, 111–112
Sickle-cell anemia, 95, 101,
    111, 327
Side-lying position, 234, 349
Sitz bath, 337
Skin
    caring for baby's,
        364–365
    changes in, 235
    darkening of, 39
    dry, itchy, 128
    peeling, in newborns, 330
    rashes, 128, 245, 330
    stretch marks on, 128, 235
Sleep, in postpartum period,
    338
Sleep disturbances, 127, 234
Sleepiness, mother's, 36
Sleeping arrangements,
    201–202
Sleeping positions
    for baby, 41, 332
    for mother, 110
Sleep patterns, newborns,
    332–333
Slings, 208
Smoking, 40–41
Snacks, 37, 78

Sneezing, in newborns, 330
Snowsuits, 214
Socks, 214
Solvents, 45–46
Sonogram, 97
Sperm, 31
Spicy foods, 49
Spina bifida, 25
Spinal anesthesia, 298,
    314–315
Spinal cord, 31–32
Spiritual Midwifery (Gaston), 169
Sponge baths, 362–363
Spontaneous abortion, 51–54
Spontaneous rupture of water
    bag, 249, 265–266, 272, 310
Stadol, 296
Startle reflex, 331
Station, 262–263
Stepping reflex, 331
Stimulant drugs, 42
Stork bites, 330
Stress, in fathers, 132–133
Stretching, 123–124, 147, 152
Stretch marks, 128, 235
Stripping of membranes, 310
Strollers, 205–206
Sucking blister, 330
Sucking reflex, 331
Sudden infant death
    syndrome (SIDS), 40,
    49, 209, 332–333
Sunscreen, 217, 359
Supplemental Nutrition
    Program for Women,
    Infants, and Children
    (WIC), 210
Support groups, 166–167, 211
Surfactant, 257
Surgical anesthetics, 83
Sushi, 63
Swaddling, 334, 360
Swallowing reflex, 331
Sweaters
    baby, 214
    maternity, 145
Swimming, 152, 253
Swimsuits, 144

Swing, 205
Swollen hands/feet, 126–127,
    146, 235–236
Syrup of ipecac, 218

T
Tailor sit/stretch, 150
Tay-Sachs disease, 101, 111
Tdap vaccine, 103
Telemetry monitors, 239, 302
Temperature taking, 346
Thalassemia major/minor,
    101, 111
Thermometer, digital, 217
Third trimester, 185–322
3-D ultrasound, 98
Three-sided sleepers, 201
Tights, 145
Toco-dynamometer, 303
Tocolytics, 173–175
Toiletries, 217–218
Tooth brushing, 50
Toothpaste, 50
Touchpoints, Birth to 3 (Brazelton
    and Sparrow), 408
Towels, 214
Toxemia, 194
Toxoplasmosis, 45, 181
Transcutaneous electrical
    nerve stimulation
    (TENS), 301
Transvaginal ultrasound, 97
Transverse position, 246, 247,
    304–305
Trimesters
    first, 29–116
    second, 117–183
    third, 185–322
    fourth, 323–368
    length of, 21
Triplets
    See also Multiples
    cesarean delivery for,
        190, 306
    hCG levels with, 34
Trisomy 18, 99, 100
Trisomy 21, 99, 100, 101
Trophoblastic tissue, 51

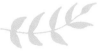

Also Available

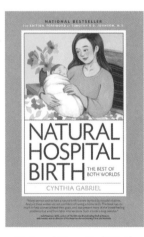

Natural Hospital Birth
978-1-55832-917-1

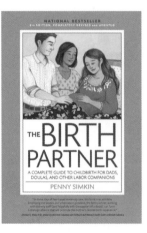

The Birth Partner
978-1-55832-910-2

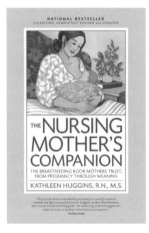

**The Nursing Mother's
Companion**
978-1-55832-882-2

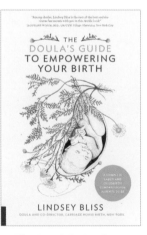

**The Doula's Guide to
Empowering Your Birth**
978-1-55832-895-2

5